SHADOW ON THE RAINBOW

Shadow on the Rainbow

on the

A Story of Faith, Hope, and Life

by

Linda Rogers McGehee

SMYTH&HELWYS
PUBLISHING, INCORPORATED • MACON, GEORGIA

Smyth & Helwys Publishing, Inc.
6316 Peake Road
Macon, Georgia 31210-3960
1-800-747-3016
©2002 by Smyth & Helwys Publishing

Library of Congress Cataloging-in-Publication Data

McGehee, Linda Rogers, 1941-
 Shadow on the rainbow : a story of friendship, hope, and life /
 by Linda Rogers McGehee.
 p. cm.
 ISBN 978-1-57312-381-5
 1. Cancer—Religious aspects—Christianity.
 2. Cancer patients—Religious life.
 I. Title.

BV4910.33M35 2002
248.8'6—dc21

                                    2002012614
                                       CIP

Contents

Part Two: Reflections

To honor Rev. Barbara Oliver
And her beloved family

Dedicated to my sister/mama Merle McMullen for believing,
and my sweet husband Leo for making all things possible

Thanks for passionate cheers of encouragement:
Scott, Teri, William, Melissa, Michael & Clay McGehee,
Peter Rogers, Donna Harding, Jerry & Ev Lee, Jan Purvis,
Becki Pickett, and Phyllis Parker

I would not give anything for the simplicity which is on the near side of complexity, but I would give everything for the simplicity which is on the far side of complexity.

—*unknown*

Foreword

"All good poems start out as a lump in the throat." What Robert Frost said concerning poetry could be said of most all other written words.

That's where the words in *Shadow on the Rainbow* got their start—as a lump in the throat of a friend who, along with others, waited with one she loved for death to come too soon. That tragic loss cast a dark shadow on many rainbows. But it eventually gave birth to this book, a book that might yet weave new rainbows of hope through many sad shadows of loss.

When Linda Rogers McGehee holds a shovel in her hand, she creates spaces for people to walk and sit and play and work. (She is a landscape artist, not unlike Elizabeth in the book!) But when she holds a pen in her hand, Linda creates a different kind of space, space for us to wonder and ponder and weep and laugh, space for us to ask God and each other and ourselves the hardest questions about the deepest pains and darkest shadows that we have to bear and face and find our way through.

Here is a book for all who have ever wept and wondered. For all who have ever grieved, here is help. For all who have ever stumbled through long nights and staggered through great loss, here is a place to sit awhile and rest awhile and listen for God, who hangs out rainbows and holds out hope, even in a weary land of deep darkness and many shadows.

Charles E. Poole
Jackson, Mississippi
Pentecost, 2001

Part One

Elizabeth

Ruth believes the old song words, "His eye is on the sparrow and I know He watches me." She says, "It's a truth worthy of trust for a lifetime." I'm pretty sure those words come from a proverb grasping at the proverbial straw and tell her, "The words are full of hope but they come with no guarantee." Its strange how Ruth and I feel so different about such things. Our backgrounds are not the same, but I just got to tell you, we were both cut out from damaged goods. Even so, Ruth is filled with faith while I tend to put my trust in the secrets of happiness that were given to me in the first stages of my childhood.

Ruth settles in and says, "Elizabeth, tell me again."

I start with the first memories. "The day Mother died all our flowers lost their bright color, even the goldfish in the lily pond just sat there, looking sad. Up until then I'd found being happy was easy. My mother shared simple secrets that make a person know exactly what to do if you want to live a happy life. We had a favorite place to sit and talk. The goldfish pond. It was there she told me everything that later saved me."

Ruth says, "Get to the part where you learned the secrets."

"Before Mother died," I say, "when the sun rose from sleep in the eastern edges of a dark sky, my father would leave for work in his blue pickup truck. Mother would reach into the kitchen cabinet and pull down a long box filled with Reese's candy, open the refrigerator and take out two Coca-Colas. We'd walk outside through the kitchen door into a canopy of oak trees filled with birds busy singing. Beyond the trees and into the sunny garden we'd take a ritual stroll, still dressed in our long white nightgowns. They'd drag damp dew as we walked barefoot through prickly green grass to the rose garden. We knew the roses by name. 'Morning, Tiny Bess. How's my pretty Tiffany today?' Mother would ask and I'd giggle. Everybody knew roses couldn't talk, but I believed they could feel. When one died another would always come to take its place. Mother would guide me along. Next we'd look for the pink carnations and breath deep their peppermint aroma. We'd always save the best viewing until last. We'd sit crossed-legged beside the fishpond. Large golden fish darted in and out of yellow water lilies. 'There's a secret to having a good life, Elizabeth,' Mother would tell me."

It was because of mother that I later came to understand pain and still care so deeply about joy. That's the flip side of double-edged knowledge. Maybe Mother didn't know that complete gladness means you can reach just as deeply into the core of life's sadness.

We'd stay by our fishpond talking. "Some people get to live long lives," Mother would say. "Others live short lives. It's not the length of life that's important, Elizabeth. How you use your life is all that really matters."

Then Mother would instruct, "Always look for beauty. It surrounds us every day." She'd take me around the pond, pointing out beauty. "See the bark on that tree?" We'd brush our fingers across its silvery roughness. "Can you believe how many different patterns butterfly wings have? Elizabeth, just *glory* in every sight. Hear those frogs? Hear that wind? Watch it make the willow dance. You can't be lonely if you cherish the sounds and smells of the earth," she'd tell me.

Some days, Mother would tell secrets. "There are two things that always bring happiness. The first is to be able to love everybody, Elizabeth." Mother taught by example. "Don't we have fun finding the things that we put in the packages we mail to your cousins every week?" she'd say. One half-cup of coffee. A bit of sugar. Some flower seeds. "It's hard times, Elizabeth, but we've got a lot of the thing you need most. You and I know how to love."

On other days by the goldfish pond Mother would tell the second way to be happy. "Elizabeth, always have something that you love doing." I was well acquainted with Mother's example of having something to do that we loved.

"We love growing flowers!" I'd shout.

Sometimes when I tell Ruth about my childhood she jumps in at some point to tell me about her own mother. "My mother was my hero," Ruth might say. Not today, though. Today, Ruth says, "Your mother gave you the secrets. But God gave her that knowledge. So, in His way, He was watching over you."

"How was a five-year-old supposed to know that?" I reply and start back telling my story. "After Mother died I went to live with my older sister and tried so hard to keep remembering the secrets for happiness. But I became a sickly child. One day at the doctor's office, I lay on a hard table weeping. What I wanted was Mother.

"Even now, talking to you, Ruth, I remember that day I'd wheezed to empty white walls and struggled for breath. The air I could grab smelled of medicine and rubbing alcohol. The old doctor had said, 'I know a place you can live that will help you feel better. This asthma that you've got requires special care.'"

"But you didn't want special care, did you?" Ruth says.

"No, I wanted my childhood. If I couldn't have that then I wanted my sister to come into that doctor's room and take Mother's place so I would have a mama. My sister answered my plea and came to comfort me. I held my arms out to her. 'You were calling me,' she told me years later.

"That's when I started calling my sister my mama," I tell Ruth.

"I don't know what God was thinking," Ruth interrupts. "Sometimes I'd like to pinch a hole in Jesus. I just hate that the same week your sister became your mama you lost her, too."

"Me and you," I say, "we keep expecting life to be fair."

"Get to the part where they send you away, Elizabeth. Tell about the circle of children."

"They sent me to live in the Preventorium in a small town near Mendenhall. The clinic connected to the TB hospital. We'd stand around in a circle drinking our daily milk at the clinic. The grass was worn thin by shuffling children's feet. The dust covered our shoes. 'Look for beauty,' Mother's voice would whisper inside my head. I'd turn my face from the circle of sad kids and watch grasshoppers play in green grass. Some days one would climb up a single blade and wait, watching me watch him. I was waiting, too. I was waiting for my life to be happy."

Ruth says, "I'd bet my bootie on that." She's religious. But it's her tendency to be irreverent I like. "Young'uns," she adds, "are suppose to be happy."

"At night we kids slept in metal beds," I continue. "The room was empty of everything except sleeping children and sound. Coughing. Crying. Whispers in the night. I'd watch the moonlight in the window near me. Every night someone cried. Not me, not me; Mother wouldn't want me to live my life crying. 'It's not me,' I'd whisper onto a damp pillow."

Ruth says, "Tell me about the train, Elizabeth."

I could always feel the train coming. The train wheels whispered, "Mis-shoo, Mis-shoo, miss you." I was wondering. . . if I jumped on the track, would it carry me closer to or further from my mama?

"Elizabeth, it wasn't a butterfly that saved you."

"Maybe, Ruth. Just maybe. That train was coming fast. There was a voice. 'Jump, jump.'"

"Elizabeth, that was not your mother's voice."

"I knew that, Ruth." The voice was near. The voice was loud. Jump! Jump! That's when the yellow butterfly with spotted wings landed on my foot. The movement from the passing train blew the hem of my dress up and around in a circle. Kind of like a dancer.

"Elizabeth, even with the noise of the train, that butterfly stayed on your toe. I'm telling you, an angel in the form of a butterfly saved you."

"Oh, Ruth, I was just a child. That butterfly held my attention till the train moved out of view."

"Mercy me, Elizabeth. Someday you'll trust your knowledge.
God is God. Seeing, feeling, proving—that's Earth-connected stuff."

Forgive me, sir,
I sure don't know
Your name.
Lord? God? Shepherd?
Meanwhile.
I
Glory
In the
Questions

Father?
Take comfort
I'm a puzzle

I
Ponder
Else
How
Can
I Dwell
Much less live
In your house
Forever.

Amen.

It's me,
Elizabeth

Chapter One

Ruth

Stoney Creek is wide in territory if narrow in outlook. When Ruth was growing up strangers, though politely welcomed, were quietly unwelcome. "Them folks, they don't bother nobody," was a high compliment, requiring years to earn.

The mountain area poverty sharply contrasted tantalizing natural beauty. Purple mountain wildflowers bowed down to early killing frost. Old time religion was spoon-fed to hungry people. Ruth's childhood preacher stressed repentance and emphasized washing away of sin through baptism. Ruth's faith was powerful, and the drama of immersion and resurrection to a new life held such fascination for her that she had herself baptized on seven different occasions.

Ruth loved the sound of words, strong saving grace pulpit words even if she did have a fondness for swearing. "If you stop saying them cuss words, I'll git ya a new dress," a deacon had offered. The promise of a new dress did not equal the fun of shocking everyone. Ruth held fast and wouldn't give up this mischievous pleasure.

She was a good little girl deeply connected to the earth. "Damn and double damn," she would say, but her innocence belied these words and was part of her charm. Tradition held that on birthdays children in the tiny mountain church were given a penny for each year of their age. On her third birthday, Ruth had walked down the aisle. She stood up front, waiting, to be given her birthday money. Other children came forth, but only Ruth asked the old preacher, "Mister, can I sing a song?"

"Praise God, yes child, you surely can sing a song." He'd removed everything off the communion table, lifted the small child on top of it. Ruth sang in a loud clear voice, "Let Others See Jesus In You."

Ruth's family lived at the foot of the mountains down Hurley Hollow. The house was small with only one bathroom for a family of five, but it stood proud and represented the good fortune of ownership.

Most of Ruth's life her family had lived in rental houses. Her brother Paul had often stayed up nights guarding Ruth after she was born. Large river rats sometimes strayed into the rental houses they'd lived in at the time of her birth. Rats that looked like small dogs. It was not until Ruth was sixteen years old that the family lived in the Hurley Hollow house. It was the first home they'd ever owned.

Across the way from the new house the kids and their mother, Maude, planted tobacco on a small, borrowed plot of land. The funds from the sale of the tobacco were used to buy something special for everyone on Christmas Day. During the year Maude washed and ironed clothes for families who could afford to have someone else do their laundry. The whole family, including Ruth's youngest sister, Robin, picked green beans for a farmer during summer months. Maude cleaned a large group of chicken houses earning funds for the family. Some of Stoney Creek's families had money. "But, most of 'em wuz about like us," Maude would later say. "I'm a-telling you, I despised that damn chicken house. It was hotter'n hell and stunk up yer clothes, Ga-awl lay!" Ruth adored her mother and referred to Maude in later years as, "my hero."

Duncan Chapel Baptist Church was the center of the Bolivar children's life. Church met every Wednesday night and three times on Sunday. Year round Ruth's family scrubbed the floors and cleaned the windows and walls until the building shone for every church service. In bitter cold winter early on Saturday mornings the family walked in snow to light the fire in the big heater, which warmed the building for Sunday services. This labor added thirty dollars a month to their income.

The church was a white wooden building sitting on top of a hillside. Whenever Ruth spied the tall steeple just above the roofline her heart was filled with happiness. She loved church; its message and its music and could be heard singing, "There's within my heart a melody. Jesus whispers sweet and low, fills my every longing, keeps me singing as I go." Music was Ruth's comfort. She sings even now, in perfect pitch, every word to any song you can name.

Ruth's enthusiasm for life originated from deep inside and she would not be deterred by the limitations of rural Tennessee. After high school she earned her bachelor's degree in education from East Tennessee State University. She became a schoolteacher at the Old Midway School where she had once been a student. "You don't have to live your whole life in Stoney Creek," Ruth often reminded herself.

One Sunday morning Ruth walked down the aisle of Duncan Chapel Baptist Church just as she had as a small child so long ago going down for her birthday pennies. The choir was singing, "Here Am I, Send Me, Lord."

"I offer you my faith today," Ruth told the church members. "I want to become an ordained minister." The room was alive with Ruth's passion but at war with her vision. Most of Stoney Creek's folks felt a woman had no business trying to preach.

Maude didn't want beloved daughter Ruth to leave home and told her, "Well, there'd be 'You Picked a Fine Time to Leave Me, Lucille'." Ruth owed seventeen hundred dollars on her new car, but she wasn't worried.

"I have a little money saved," she told her family, "I have a lot of faith inside me."

Some of the mountain people believed Ruth had a genuine call from God. It was those people of understanding who mailed the unsolicited checks that paved the way for Ruth to enter Southern Baptist Theological Seminary in Louisville, Kentucky.

"Sometimes I'd need a certain amount of money and on that very day, the exact amount of money needed would arrive in the mail," Ruth later recalled.

Funds were not the only deterrent to Ruth's goal. In the seminary women who wanted to be ministers faced the traditional Baptist assumption that God ordained men to lead the church. Ruth overlooked their smugness, made close seminary friendships that would last her whole life, worked hard, and relied on faith. With diligence, and being no stranger to hard work, Ruth earned a Master of Divinity degree in mid-1985.

Stoney Creek's simple mountain folks were not impressed.

"Ruth is going to talk to us today," some would say when she visited her home in Stoney Creek.

"I reckon she is some kind of missionary or somethin," others would explain.

"Huh, I wouldn't walk across the street to hear no woman preach," you could hear up and down the hollows.

Ruth's sister Robin would fuss, "Shoot, round here folks think women should stay home, have young'uns, maybe be school teachers; but don't dare be nothing else, though."

But Ruth loved God. She held fast the cherished memories of the morning's sunlight reaching through the windows of the Duncan Chapel Baptist Church and a Bible with its edges worn from wear and left wide open. She loved the fresh flowers, cut from fields nearby and placed with care on top of the altar table. She'd found comfort in the anticipation of a collection plate serenely waiting. Piano music had filled the church and lifted the spirit of the people seated on the pews. It had been a safe place where happiness and hope seemed to share space. There was not one thing about Ruth's childhood church that caused fear or sadness. It had been a place of peace and preparation for Ruth. She loved its people.

No one could have known the sorrow the future held for Ruth, her cherished mother, brother, and sister. Paul believed that each family member was part of what he called, "the body of their family" and often said, "I think of myself as the legs or backbone, but Ruth is the heart." The family who had lived through so much still had a great challenge left to face.

Praise somersaults
On
Mountain green.

And
Four leaf clover

With
Birds singing.
Church bells ringing

Calling me.
Work or play?

I love each day.
I know
You.

Amen.

Your friend
Ruth

Chapter Two

There Is No One Like You

Faith is a constant struggle for me, but Ruth's faith is so strong that it led her away from her mountain home in Tennessee to the center of Mississippi. Ruth is the only female Baptist minister in our state, and I'm proud that our church is wide open to the idea of women in the ministry. The day I first saw Ruth I didn't even have a clue about the joy she would bring into my life, much less anticipate the sorrow.

North Church is Baptist in form, but unlike most Southern Baptist churches here, our choir processes and recesses with our ministers following and wearing long black clerical robes. The church building has no stained-glass windows. "Don't close out the world; bring the world inside," the church building architect had been told. A cross hanging on a church wall is common in Episcopal or Catholic churches, but unusual in Baptist churches. We like our simple, large wooden cross hanging above a several-hundred-thousand-dollar Austin Organ, donated in memory of one of our members. The church encourages having female deacons as well as male. People say our church is more New Testament than Old Testament. Ruth's little mountain church would appreciate the spirit of our church, but they'd question its lack of Southern tradition.

When I first joined this affluent church, I had been afraid of finding a place for myself, but Ruth seemed confident of her spot from her very first day. She walked down the aisle wearing white sandals underneath a black clergy robe. White sandals before Easter and under black.

Good God! I'd thought.

Ruth followed the choir, moving in procession down the aisle. Gracefully, in the unexpected but lovely way large women sometimes move. Her yellow hair reflected shining light against the solemn black robe. Most anyone could have told you, but I knew right off the bat that mischievousness danced around her bright red mouth. Supreme confidence radiated out of blue eyes as calm as morning glories growing beside a country roadside.

A few days later I went to the church office to introduce myself to Ruth and she made me mad. "Hello, I'm Elizabeth," I began.

Ruth barked at me, "Elizabeth, I've been told you're the person I need to call to get fresh pine straw placed in the children's playground. How soon can you get it done? Those young'uns are getting eaten up by red ants. When can you do something about that, too?"

I never got around to saying that I had stopped by to tell her I'd been picked to be her special Caregiver. "By gosh, the new minister sure is bossy," I told the church secretary and went home thinking how interesting things were going to get watching this bold young woman fit into our church membership with its illusion of sophistication and wealth. Much of our congregation is educated, professional. Not me, of course. I got married too young to get much education. We're a church of doctors, lawyers, and congressmen who dress to fit our roles. I'm a landscape contractor. But in our membership are one former city Mayor, a Gubernatorial, and a U.S. Senator.

Did I tell you I'm a landscape contractor? I'm talented. It oozes. North Church loves talent. My mother could stick a broomstick in the ground and it'd sprout flowers. I was too young to remember much about her but the flowers. My own love of them keeps me close to her even after her death all those years ago. People in our church like the way I bring nature into a part of our worship service with my flowers on the church altar.

Our membership is in touch with the heartbeat of the city, too. Most of us sit on important charitable boards that make a real difference in folks' lives. We're big on encouraging lay members to make the important decisions about church polity. One thing we treasure is our very formal, elegant worship services. Where will Ruth of the White Sandals fit?

In time, Ruth and I became friends. I'd tease, "I thought you were a first-class witch the first time I met you." That thought has since changed. Whenever I see her, she greets me with a "Hi, honey" and a big hug. Ruth loves me. I'm almost old enough—not quite—to be her mother, but Ruth is ageless.

We're movie buddies. I closed my eyes through most of *Jurassic Park*. Ruth never blinked. We eat out together. Ruth has to diet. I don't. Mostly we share ideas. It's our big thing. "Let's visit," Ruth will say. We're laughers. I make Ruth giggle. We swap childhood stories.

"My Mommy taught me that sin is like soot on snow," Ruth might say.

"I crawled under the house the day Mother died," I might answer, "to count the camellias she had been rooting under overturned jelly jars."

Soon after Ruth came to our church, we found ourselves forgetting any shallow illusions we held of ourselves. Stiff services help me keep God at a safe distance. Ruth and our senior minister are tending toward less formal and more passionate services. Ruth's comfort with who she is and where she came from is helping me move along on my spiritual journey and get on with *getting over myself.* Her humanity lifts spirits. Ruth sees past personal veneer, looks into a person's heart, and finds a spirit's potential. She calls it forth and leads the members down paths that help develop each one's own potential for lay ministry in the world. She's also become pastoral director of mission trips that lead us from Kentucky to New York to Chicago.

Children are Ruth's special interest. It's not unusual to hear her singing to them, "There is no one exactly like you. You can search the whole world over, but there is no one exactly like you." She works with kids of all races in our city. She loves the children in the inner city areas as dearly as she loves the children of our own church.

Ruth's been here at North Church for four years. Maude, Paul, and Ruth's sister Robin often visit and our church family adores the unique qualities of Ruth's family. Especially Ruth's mother, Maude, and her wonderful mountain-poet voice. One Sunday after lunch at the city's largest country club, Maude whispered to Ruth, "Oh, my Lordy . . . nobody paid."

No one anticipated the extremely high price tag about to be placed on our happiness.

I'm where I started
Stuck
Running fast forward.

Dragging
Past.

Slow Breath
Dear Heart.

If I
Get it together

Will you
Carry some part?

Amen.

It's me,
Elizabeth

Chapter Three

Is God More God When Things Go Good?

Bad news arrives at a place that seems natural for disaster. Myrtle Beach is not a white-sand, blue-water vacation haven. It is too commercial. The sand is coarse, so hard you can drive a car across it. The ringing of my family's hotel telephone can be heard over the sound of turbulent waters brushing hard rock.

"Elizabeth," the caller says, "Reverend Ruth Bolivar has been diagnosed with chronic myelocytic leukemia."

"Oh, dear God. Please, no. No!"

I phone Ruth immediately.

"I am going to lean heavily on you because you are one of the few people I know who can take this sort of thing," Ruth tells me. "My family will not be able to bear the idea that I have cancer. You will be called to help me do what I must do."

"I'm strong, Ruth. I'll be there no matter what," I say with far more confidence than I feel.

As soon as I can get back to Mississippi, Ruth comes to my home. We sit on the sofa in a room that normally shouts joy with its lighthearted furnishings. "I am afraid," she tells me. "There's so much feeling of loss. I wanted to marry someday. This means I will not be able to bear a child. I wanted to have babies! Even if I live I will never be able to have them. There are so many things left that I want to do. Why, why?"

I have no answers. My life has taught me that even the inexperienced young can't count on anything.

As the months begin to pass, Ruth starts saying, "The medicine makes me so sick and weak. What am I going to do? The doctor says that at best, I can live only a few years on this medicine."

In time Ruth comes to believe that her only hope is a bone marrow transplant. "I am trying to decide what is the best hope for my life. I am not ready to die. I want to live my life," she cries. "Even with a bone marrow transplant I only have a thirty percent chance to live." Ruth's voice sometimes is broken with grief. "If I am going to have a transplant, it has to be done in the first year of diagnosis."

"We will be there for you whatever decision you make," I promise.

When she chooses the brave path, her friends and family set about making it happen. "I just know Robin or Paul's bone marrow will be a perfect match for me," Ruth tells us with strong conviction.

Sadly, when the results come in from the blood work the doctor tells Ruth, "Your siblings are a perfect match for one another, but neither one's marrow matches yours." That limits the chance for survival from a transplant even more. Beginnings of panic and sadness form hard lines around Ruth's eyes.

Local newspapers start writing feature articles about her struggle. Our church holds a bone marrow drive. Ruth leads us into joining the national register for bone marrow transplants. We have no bone marrow match for Ruth, but we could be available to give someone else a chance at life if our bone marrow matched theirs.

Ruth's mother affectionately nicknames one of Ruth's friends "Sugarbaker." Maude says, "She reminds me of them women on TV. Designing Women." Sugarbaker and another friend that Maude calls Tess have come up with the idea that the church should hold a fund-raiser to help cover Ruth's expenses.

"This will give our church the opportunity for everyone to be a part of Ruth's journey," says our senior minister.

"I hate the idea of public exposure to my private self," Ruth tells me.

I know Ruth doesn't relish pity. I know she's coming to grips with the terror of the possibility of losing her life. While Ruth gathers courage to face the pain and eventualities that lie before her, she has to deal with private, personal issues.

"I don't want pity. I'm not used to receiving help. I like giving help."

There is a constant search for matching bone marrow. We all believe it is out there . . . somewhere.

"Elizabeth, how could there be not one bone marrow that matches mine?" Ruth asks. Fear locks into our hearts.

The children of the church start praying for a miracle. I'm not sure children need to believe in miracles.

We all know time is running out.

The answering machine light flashes a bright, red light when I enter my house one day. I press the button for messages. Ruth's voice sings out, "Elizabeth, I am going to get French marrow! Call me. The donor lives in Paris. Just think, in this whole wide world, there is someone just for me." She's laughing in a happy voice.

Who is God
To lost children
People in pain, afraid
Sick or weary?

Is God
More God
When things go good?

I shout out
Heal!

Nothing
Happens

Never has
Never will

I give in
Give up
Sulking around

Look down
In prayer

Look up
In peace

At last
You're here.

Amen.

Trying to be,
Elizabeth

Chapter Four

Daughter Be Confident

As Ruth waits for a transplant date, her medication and illness bring on enormous fatigue.

"I'm tired, and I feel so weak. I'm supposed to speak this Sunday. I'm not sure I have enough energy. I have half a mind to call in someone else to do the sermon," Ruth says one Tuesday.

"You don't have to make yourself preach Sunday if you don't feel like it. Get someone else," I reply, totally unaware that the sermon might be important to Ruth and to me.

Thursday afternoon Ruth goes into her office and closes the door. When she comes out, she has written Sunday's sermon. "Chances Are," she calls it. It is typed and ready for the Sunday service.

On Sunday, Maude, Paul, and Robin are in town. They seat themselves on an end aisle and wait for Ruth to speak. The lay reader reads from the Bible about the woman who touches Jesus' robe and is healed. I hear the words, *a woman who had a problem with blood.* I tense up. Suddenly, I feel frightened. I wish I had asked Ruth what she planned to say. A low, soft voice begins singing. I am disoriented. Singing? Where did the sound come from?

"I must tell Jesus all of my troubles," the voice sings.

I look up, and Ruth is walking toward the pulpit . . . singing. Has she lost her mind? Is the illness too much to bear? I worry.

Ruth takes her rightful place and continues singing. "I cannot bear these burdens alone." Ruth leans over the pulpit and delivers the entire sermon as though she were the woman who touched

Jesus' garment and was healed. She speaks as though she is that very woman. "As I watched from a pretty far distance, I felt my courage beginning to grow. The anticipation within me started to churn. My hope rose like the waves in the sea beyond. And just as I was about to yell out, 'Hey, Jesus! Look at me, notice me,' a man came and fell at Jesus' feet and started begging . . ."

Oh, my goodness, I think. *Ruth is begging God to heal her!*

She's saying, "I'll have to say, I was surprised, and I was disappointed as Jesus turned to go with the man. 'What's the use?' I cried to myself, 'things never work out for people like me!'"

Too hard, I think, and cry open tears as I listen to Ruth speak.

"The tassel of His prayer shawl was within sight, and in a flash, I reached my hand around the waist of the beggar in front of me. I reach for that part of His garment! I didn't care if *He* noticed me or not. It was healing I was after, and if I had to steal that blessing, then so be it!

"'Who touched me?' Jesus asked. I was consumed with my needs, my wants, my condition, my issues. And so, I blurted it all out. I told the truth, and then I waited for judgment to fall. Do you know what Jesus did? You read the account in the Bible this morning. But I love to repeat it. He said to me, 'Daughter, be confident. Your faith has made you well!'"

If only Ruth could be well, I sit there thinking. In the days to come, Ruth's sermon stays in my mind, and I begin understanding something I've never understood. It is about some need I've longed for all my life. I was five when mother died. My own young father had lacked the gift of fathering. After living in the Preventorium and after a year's stay with Daddy's brother and wife, my older sister took me into her home to live and gave me much love. But her husband was so emotionally ill that he had trouble loving his own daughter. He could not love me. I grew up desperately wanting to hear a father call me, "Daughter!" Over the weeks I decide to claim the words from Ruth's sermon and place them in the context of my own need.

"Daughter, be confident. Your faith has made you well!"

Trees

Utterly naked in winter's shade
Hold promise

Flowers in spring
Fruit in summer

Thank you

Help me

Trust your presence
In the world

Amen.

Elizabeth

Chapter Five

Good Luck and
I Love You

Sugarbaker is holding a party for Ruth's thirty-sixth birthday. For my gift I've had my neighbor make a huge poster with the bodies of "All the Great Blondes of the World" and superimposed the face of Ruth on each and every one of them. Ruth as Madonna. Ruth as Marilyn Monroe. But I feel unconnected to the laughter and gaiety at the party. It might be Ruth's last birthday.

Ruth's love of life demands a chance. The "French Marrow," as we call it, seems to be that opportunity. What I don't know is that Ruth's doctor here has not encouraged her to have the transplant. Ruth believes the transplant is her only chance to live a full life and is preparing to leave Mississippi, go home, and then enter Emory Hospital in Atlanta to receive the marrow transplant. Now Sugarbaker has us busy making plans for a farewell party in Ruth's honor.

Springtime in the South brings azaleas, dogwoods, and redbuds. I've filled the church's great hall with flowers and huge balloons. Children of the church have made posters signed with "Good luck" and "I love you."

At the farewell party, the fear that had seemed to loom so near me at the birthday party subsides. I join in the great fun and feeling of celebration. The French Marrow will mean life for our friend.

Sugarbaker surprises Ruth with a visit from an Elvis impersonator. He's good. We sing and yell. "Elvis! Elvis!" Ruth's up front sitting on a throne-like chair. Balloons tied with brightly-colored ribbon dance over her head. Everyone joins in when "Elvis" sings all of his hits. It's my era of music, but Ruth knows and sings every word with him. She blushes and hams it up. Ruth, secure in the knowledge that the needed bone marrow had been located, joins in the fun. She plays her part so well that at one point Elvis says, "Ca, ca, cool it baby, after all, we is in a church."

God

Only you know
The inside
Of a
Child kneeling
In prayer

You touch
Sharp-edged stars
Volcano depths
Height of sky

I want to trust your vision
I'm ill-equipped to follow
Where you go

Light my way.

Amen.

It's me,
Elizabeth

Chapter Six

Could Ruth Get a Miracle?

Ruth is at home in Stoney Creek with her family for a month before she enters the hospital to have the transplant. I keep trying to withdraw emotionally in hopes of protecting myself from all that is coming. It doesn't work. Fear just eats at my bones as the appointed time for Ruth to enter the hospital approaches. Paul keeps us posted on the waiting and writes in his formal manner, "Ruth's determination and bravery continue to be a good example to each of us. She remains steadfast in her optimism of the bone marrow procedure, however the waiting and postponements have been excruciating . . ."

Lack of available space in the hospital causes further delay. Ruth and I talk on the phone and make plans for her to meet me in Charlotte, North Carolina, and visit my family, but the hospital calls saying that they are now ready for her. Our plans are canceled. Ruth and Robin go to Atlanta to get ready to enter Emory Hospital.

Her sister has made what they call a bargain with Ruth. Robin said, "I'll put my life on hold and stay with you and help you every way possible. You do your part, and together we will get through this transplant."

Paul worries about Ruth and Robin. Robin's job has been steady employment, not easy to come by in the mountains. The job provides health insurance coverage for Robin and her sons. What if the leave of absence she's taken makes her lose her job?

Maude wants to stay with Ruth in the hospital, but Ruth insists, "You stay home and take care of Robin's boys. I'm counting on you. Someone has to take care of my Cleo."

Cleo, Ruth's dog, is a gift from Robert, Ruth's best friend from seminary days. Cleo is her baby. Every night Ruth sings to Cleo, "I love you, Cleo, oh yes I do, I love you, Cleo, oh yes I do."

"Mommy," Ruth tells Maude, "I'm counting on you to feed Cleo and see she gets plenty of affection while I'm getting the transplant."

We all get a good laugh when Maude responds in typical Maude fashion, "Well, piss on the dog." But of course she will do what her children asked of her. Maude stays in Stoney Creek. Praying for her child. She's put her faith and trust in a God who has always been there for her family.

Paul calls to say, "All nine of us have crowded into a two-bedroom Atlanta apartment loaned to Ruth by a family of North Church. Ruth has insisted we be together this last night. It's something we're all glad to do for her."

Sugarbaker has the bright idea to take her family to Atlanta the day before Ruth is to enter the hospital. Sugarbaker's husband goes to a ballgame while all the others go together to Six Flags.

"Who on earth but Ruth," I wonder, "would want to go to Six Flags over Georgia the day before they enter a hospital to have a bone marrow transplant?"

Robin hates fast-moving, high-flying carnival rides, but anytime she refuses to ride on one Ruth pretends to look really sad and says, "But you've got to ride what I say because I have leukemia."

Robin jokes, "I'm getting tired of this cancer crap."

Paul later writes to the church, "It was so difficult to leave them when they entered the hospital the next day. After a tearful embrace, none of us wanted to let go of each other. In the days following, I've been unable to get Ruth off my mind for longer than a few minutes at a time."

Ruth's preparation treatment for the transplant seems to be going well. There are no visible side effects, only anxiety over what Ruth faces. But then on Sunday Ruth has an allergic reaction to one of the chemotherapy treatments. She has chills, vomiting, diarrhea, and hives. By Monday she improves some as they slow the dosage of chemo and give her Benadryl to offset the allergy. She's scheduled to begin high-dosage radiation on Monday along with chemo.

Paul is trying to work and longing to be with his sisters. He calls to say, "By noon I told my colleagues at work that I had to leave and that I would be in touch. My wife Ann helped me pack and assured me that she and our daughter Beth would be okay. I left in mid-afternoon for Atlanta. Ruth was very tired and in a weakened state so I stayed with her during the evening. There was nothing that I could do to help her but give moral support. We drew strength from each other and I was less anxious knowing that I could reach out and touch her when I needed to. Robin is such a marvelous caregiver for Ruth. She remains at her side constantly and never complains. No sacrifice is too great for our beloved sister . . ."

Ruth is transported to the Veteran Administration Hospital for the high dosage of radiation therapy twice each day. The immediate side effects include a burning sensation in her esophagus, extreme fatigue, and nausea. "We try not to think about the long-term effect the radiation might cause or organ damage or hair loss or many other things that we perhaps haven't imagined," Robin says.

Ruth has developed a fondness for the kind and gentle radiologist, Dr. Keller, who is fascinated that Ruth is an ordained Baptist minister. He brings her the poem, "Ordination" by James Autry about the moving ordination of a woman into the ministry. When Dr. Keller comments to Ruth that she seems so serene in the face of this very difficult challenge, Ruth informs him, "We have undergone many emotional difficulties throughout our lives and this is only one more obstacle. God will be faithful as we endure it."

I fax little short stories to Ruth as a way of keeping up with her every few days, signing them, "Don't you let go sweet gal . . . hold on; we love and need you. Love to you from 'Hey, Honey.'"

A few days before the transplant is to take place, Robin calls saying that Ruth wants me to come to Atlanta.

"Remind Ruth that I've made plans to be in Atlanta on Thursday with the group coming to be with her for the transplant," I tell her.

I can hear Ruth wail in the background when Robin relays the message. "Do not wait," she shouts. "I need to see you now."

I reassure her, "Tell Ruth don't worry, I don't know if it will be by horse or by train, but I am on my way. I'll see her no later than tomorrow morning." I cancel an appointment and by midnight I am doing exactly what my husband asked me not to do: driving around Atlanta searching for a room in which to spend the night.

The next morning when I enter Ruth's hospital room I am shocked to see how ill she looks. I sit quietly as Ruth sleeps. When she wakes, I hold her, my arms around her as she weeps and tells me how angry she is feeling. "I came to the hospital feeling well and look how sick they've made me with these treatments."

I remember that when I was giving birth to my first son, there had been times when the pain felt so intense that I couldn't remember why I was going through such pain. I beg Ruth, "Try to remember that they are not doing this to hurt you, but to save your life. It's like childbirth—sometimes it hurts so badly you forget what the pain will bring. Remember you are moving toward the beautiful life that lies before you." *Lord,* I quietly pray, *what if we are wrong and Ruth dies?*

She calms down and sleeps some more. When she wakes up she insists on getting out of bed and sitting on the sofa with me. "Let's visit," she says. I assume the role of church gossip and tell her about any news that I can remember.

"Have you been to any good movies while I've been gone?" she asks.

"It's been the worst summer for movies," I tell her. "You haven't missed one good film." I chatter and try really hard to connect her with a life that doesn't involve death.

When I leave to go home, Robin tells me, "Ruth will be all right, I just know it. We'll get our miracle."

I realize miracles don't seem to happen. It scares me to know Robin believes and is counting on one. Could Ruth get a miracle? If anyone ever needed a miracle, then certainly Ruth—so young, so needful of life—needs one. The children of our church are counting on a miracle. How will they feel when one doesn't come? Even I have hope. Maybe? The social worker has flown to France to be there when the bone marrow is harvested. It won't be long now, just a few days until the transplant. Will there be new life for Ruth?

God

Power
Beyond
Comprehension.

I believe what I see

Stars
Flowers
Wind in trees
Reflect Your Presence

Why trust sorrow?

Amen.

Elizabeth

Chapter Seven

Overwhelming Thirst

The intensive steroid treatments meant to kill Ruth's natural immune system so it won't attack the new marrow make her emotions accelerate. She's suffering heart palpitations, shortness of breath, nausea. She can't sleep. All this combined with extreme anticipation drives many bone marrow transplant patients near the edge. Ruth, though, is confident in the midst of a desperate illness. Somewhere in France a woman is preparing to enter a hospital to donate the needed marrow that must reach Ruth within twenty-four hours after harvesting. The tension is excruciating.

Ruth has lost so much of her golden hair that she asks Ernest, one of her nurses, to cut it all close to the scalp. "Have a close look," Ruth tells everyone. "Call Robert and confirm that I am a true blonde, even at the roots. Some best friend he is—always telling me what a great dye job I've got."

A group arrives at the hospital from North Church and is given sterile white masks to wear when they are in Ruth's room. Sugarbaker gets an inspiration. "Y'all, let's draw huge smiling lips on them before we go inside." Ruth howls when she sees the bright red lipstick smiles.

"Ruth continues to keep her sense of humor and very pleasant personality," says Paul.

Sugarbaker produces videotape with various church members' greetings to Ruth. She loves the church's ingenuity in choosing methods of communication, including one family who's making it possible for her to use e-mail from her hospital room. But she has been too ill most of the time to use it.

Ruth asks Sugarbaker to bring her video camera so that she can send a message back to church friends. Two nights earlier, Ruth, wide-awake, unable to sleep, wrote a poem to North Church people. She wants to read it to them on the video and conduct a tour of her room via camera for the children in the congregation. Ruth carefully explains the monitors and IVs connected to her body in a manner that won't scare them. She holds up a toothbrush made of sponges, explaining that the hospital had given it to her since brushes might cause infection. She asks the children, "Don't you think it would be more fun if I just didn't have to brush my teeth?" She doesn't tell them what we all know. Her mouth is full of raw ulcers and a thick white yeast-like substance. Ruth takes off her hat and points her bald head to the camera, saying, "My brother Paul says, 'Now you look just like Madonna.'"

In the middle of the filming, a noticeably excited young woman suddenly opens the door. Ruth introduces her as Polly O'Brien, the Emory Bone Marrow Transplant Coordinator. Ms. O'Brien announces, "I am back from France. Everything went well. The bone marrow from the French donor will be ready between midnight and one o'clock!" Less than twenty-four hours after being harvested from the young mother of two living in faraway France, the bone marrow is ready to be given to Ruth.

Paul drives the church friends to a motel to check in for the night before they all go out to eat. At such a late hour they find only a Waffle House open, but they are too hungry and much too excited about the transplant to care.

After eating, they come back to the hospital. Robin and Paul spend some private time with their beloved sister. Ruth then asks to speak to each of her waiting friends, one at a time. One, then another enters Ruth's room. They come back to the waiting room teary-eyed and visibly shaken. One says, "I tried to lead a prayer, but Ruth did it herself saying. 'Now I lay me down to sleep. I pray the Lord my soul to keep. If I should die before the marrow make, I pray the Lord my soul to take.'"

When it is time for the transplant, there is none of the drama we expected. The hospital personnel simply place it in an IV and let Ruth have anyone she wants in the room with her. She takes the French marrow in her hands and says, "This is my life, right here. My physical life is in this bag. As I drift off to sleep at some point this night, I am going to imagine that the marrow is a great ocean entering my body, going deeply, deeply into the cave of my bone and that all of it will stay and begin to grow and make new cells to replace all those that were too weak to fight. This is my challenge."

Ruth starts us singing softly an old hymn. It is like the kind she sang in her childhood church, except Ruth adds a new last line:

Softly and tenderly Jesus is calling, calling for you and for me,
See on the portals He's waiting and watching, watching for you
     and for me.
Why should we tarry when Jesus is pleading, pleading for you and
     for me!
Why should we linger and hear not His mercies, mercies for you
     and for me?

Come home, come home, ye who are weary come home.
Earnestly, tenderly Jesus is calling, Oh marrow come home!

Paul comments afterward, "No one talked—we didn't have to. God revealed himself in his servant, Ruth."

I can't help marveling at the journey of faith that has begun in a small congregation in Jackson, Mississippi, spread around the world to the marrow of a French donor in Paris, and come back full circle here in Atlanta where our beloved Ruth waits to be healed.

God of hope

Are you here
When I doubt?

You're easy to find
In the middle of green pasture
Fields of flowers

Blue sky.

I can pick a violet
And believe

In you.

It's those dry spells
When the winds blow too hard
And the sun beats down

When my cup is empty
An overwhelming thirst
Keeps me
From
You.

It's me,
Elizabeth

Chapter Eight

Crucial Days

Each night as Ruth struggles to survive the crucial first hundred days of her bone marrow transplant, I draw a line on my calendar. Ruth has made it one more day.

On the thirty-fifth day, the telephone rings. A frightened Sugarbaker says, "Elizabeth, Ruth's bilirubin count is up; she may have graft-versus-host disease in her liver! If the liver fails, Ruth can't live."

My hand grips the telephone, my worst fears realized. "Oh, my God! Sugarbaker, get prepared. We'll need to get to Atlanta. Fast."

"I'll call Tessie right now."

Shaken, too panicked to cry, I jump when the phone rings again. It's Robin, "Elizabeth, have you been told?"

"Sugarbaker's just called me. Robin, what do you want me to do?"

"Ruth says, 'get to Atlanta quick, we need you.'"

"Tell Ruth I love her. I'll be there before the day is over."

At noon, eyes red from tears that will not stop falling, I drive over to the church to meet Sugarbaker and Tessie and make reservations for our flight to Atlanta. By eleven o'clock that night, in a near state of panic, we arrive and soon are at Emory Hospital talking to Ruth's brother and sister.

Paul, relieved that we are here, says, "If you want to, you can see Ruth. She's sleeping."

Sugarbaker and Tessie decide to wait until morning, but I want to let Ruth know we have arrived. "I want to sit by her bedside for a while." Paul nods and leads me to Ruth's room.

Glad to be near Ruth, I sit on the sofa. She seems to be sleeping hard. Is she dreaming? I wonder. Silence fills the room. After a few moments she opens one eye, too exhausted, too drugged to wake fully. I whisper, "Ruth, we love you, we're here, we won't leave you."

Sitting in the dark room beside Ruth's hospital bed I hear a prayer repeat itself over and over inside my head. "Lord, be with Ruth. Let me speak the right words. Wisdom, God. Help me to have the wisdom to use the right words to be helpful. Why do I, who so often fail to believe in the power of prayer, find myself praying? Wisdom, Lord, I need wisdom."

After a while Ruth fully wakes up, fixes firm eyes on mine, and asks, "Elizabeth, do *you* think I'm going to die?" There is no doubt in my mind Ruth still wants to believe she will live.

I take her hand, give it a quick kiss, "Ruth, I am afraid. This is scary, but when I'm with you I have a strong feeling of *life*. I still believe that you are going to live."

She gives me a grateful smile and falls right back to sleep. The joy of that smile lingers heavy on my heart. I've told the truth—Ruth is full of life—and at the same moment I've lied to my friend. I do not believe she will live. Is it me who is not ready, as well as Ruth, who cannot bear to face what she must know is coming?

Later, when I leave her room, Paul is standing outside Ruth's door. In the dim hallway he looks frightened. Damp perspiration glistens on his forehead. "Someone told me I might have to tell Ruth that it is OK for her to die," he says.

"Yes," I respond without hesitation. "That time may come and it will be the thing for you to say. But Paul, that time hasn't come yet. If and when it does, you will know she's dying and that it's time to tell her to let go. You'll be able to do what you need to do." Later I wonder where the authority to say such strong words came from and then remember my prayers for wisdom. Is God here with us? Did He answer my prayer, or did my prayer sharpen my thoughts, bringing quite naturally the needed words to my mouth at the required moment?

Later Sugarbaker, Tessie, and I leave the hospital to find a place to spend the night. We came to Atlanta by jet but it takes a police car to get us to a motel. The hospital shuttle drops us off at the wrong motel, it's after midnight, and there are no available rooms. A flustered Sugarbaker flags down a passing police car. "I've got two friends across the street," she tells the officer, then suddenly realizes the policeman could misunderstand her intent. Her mouth opens and closes, gasping for breath. She slows down, carefully explaining our situation. The policeman offers to give us a ride to the right motel. Sugarbaker and Tessie crawl into the backseat of the police car as readily as if they'd been in one often. I panic. "No way," I insist, "I'm not getting into the backseat of anybody's car that has a cage built around it." Doubtful, but what can I do? Sugarbaker and Tessie are already securely seated.

I crawl into the front seat of the squad car, shut the door, and hear the police radio blaring, "There's a suspicious looking man with green hair prowling around."

"I have to check out this call before I can take you ladies to the motel," the cop informs us.

Not now, I think. I don't want to go on a police search in downtown Atlanta at two o'clock in the morning looking for some nutcase with a rainbow hairdo. The last time my husband saw me I was safe at home in Jackson, Mississippi. Now, I'm in a police car in Atlanta, prowling around for some greasy-haired hooligan.

"I hope Edwin finds the note I left on the kitchen table," I blurt out. "I told him, 'Ruth's in trouble and we've gone to Atlanta.'" If my husband closed his eyes and could see me now, right now, this very minute, he'd have a heart attack.

The officer guns the engine, racing up and down the street in hot pursuit of green hair. Thank goodness we can't find the felon. Mercifully, the officer gives up the chase and I settle down, realizing there is no other choice. Soon enough, we finally get shelter for the night.

The next day we awaken from a restless sleep and head back to the hospital. Ruth's thickened tongue makes speech difficult but she seems to feel better. She asks me, "How are your grandchildren?"

I tell her, "Great, William's so sweet; Melissa's been singing a new song. Want to hear the words?"

"Sing them to me!"

"All I really need is a song in my heart, food in my belly, love in my family."

"I love that song! Melissa made it up, I just know she did," Ruth insists. "That song sounds just *like* Melissa."

These precious moments of shared small talk don't last long. Ruth's feeling better doesn't last. Her bilirubin continues to climb. Ruth's esophagus is badly damaged from high dosages of radiation used to destroy her natural immune system. Now her own body has attacked and is trying to destroy the new bone marrow perceiving it as alien. Ruth is in terrible pain. We can only offer support. I struggle to appear calm and wring my hands and watch. Ruth draws more into herself.

Tessie and Sugarbaker seem to take better, more detached control of their emotions. Their calm, efficient action makes me less sure of myself. I stand back, glad not to be in charge.

Ruth's pain, the knowledge that she will probably die, seems to take hold of the deepest core of my own self-confidence. For once in our friendship I am lost and bewildered when I am near her. I want so badly to change the force of her failing heath, and I can hardly bear that our golden friend is not going to get to live out her glittering future.

Paul calls his wife. "Things are looking real bad. You better bring Mommy and Robin's boys to Atlanta."

They arrive in the night. We wait to see if Ruth's liver will recover. It continues to fail. Now all of Ruth's family is near her.

Closer to the weekend, Sugarbaker and Tessie feel they need to get home to their young children. "If Ruth is dying," Tessie says, "our kids are going to need us to be with them."

"I just don't think I can bring myself to leave Ruth. Especially when she wants me to stay," I tell them.

"We are going to have to realize," Tessie says, "Ruth may not be able to use good judgment right now. You know the medication and her illness may cloud her judgment."

"I don't care. I'm sure Ruth's judgment is impaired, but as long as she asks me to stay I can't bring myself to leave her." Tessie's sureness sometimes throws me. She always seems to know just what to do. I always see several possibilities. I don't want to be practical, but more than that I want to respond the way Ruth wants me to respond.

"Would you ask Ruth how she feels about us returning to Jackson on Saturday?" Tessie and Sugarbaker ask me.

I make myself do it. "Ruth, Tessie and Sugarbaker think it is about time for them to get home to their girls. How would you feel about us going home this weekend?"

"Do not leave!"

"Don't worry," I say. "I understand what you are telling me." She is afraid that if we leave she'll die.

That afternoon after Ruth's mother, Maude, and Robin's sons arrive and have been at the hospital for a while, we take them to lunch as a diversion from the stress. Maude, getting a big kick out of Sugarbaker's driving skills, says, "You drive just like Ruth."

"Yep, I'm good at this driving," Sugarbaker says and makes a U-turn right in the middle of Peachtree Street.

"Oh, my God," I say and close my eyes.

Elaborating, Maude tells Sugarbaker, "Whenever I fuss at Ruth about the way she drives, she always says, 'Don't worry, I've got Jesus in the car with me!' I tell her, 'Well, if you don't be more careful you are going to get Him killed.'" It feels good to be able to find something to laugh about for a few moments.

After lunch we go back to the hospital, and Ruth asks Tessie to do guided imagery with her. I watch as Tessie begins by asking Ruth, "What do you want to work on first?"

Ruth says, "I want the new bone marrow to be accepted by my body."

Tessie asks, "How do you visualize this new bone marrow?"

"It is blue in color and shaped like fancy L's," Ruth replies. "Remember, we are dealing with French marrow! My cells are white and oblong."

Tessie begins talking in a soft voice. "I want you to think about these blue cells as a brave army coming out to help your body heal." She speaks directly to the white oblong cells. "These blue cells are not unfriendly—they are here to make you stronger. Welcome them and make them your friend. Do not be afraid of them. Take them into your body and let them become a part of you. Watch these white oblong cells—they are becoming a soft blue as they begin to realize the L-shaped cells are not the enemy." Tessie continues to speak, and with time, Ruth falls into a deep and restful sleep.

Later, when a nurse tries to draw blood from of the tubes that are attached to Ruth's chest, the blood refuses to flow. Ruth, in pain and frustration, has wedged her body across the bed sideways. I stand with my hands holding her head, Sugarbaker holds her feet, and Tessie holds her hand from one side and tries using the imaging to relax Ruth's body. The nurse hovers over us, desperately trying to draw the needed blood, which will not flow without cooperation from Ruth's body. At that moment, the notion of the Holy Trinity takes on new meaning to me. A cross is formed by the position of Ruth's body. It feels as though we are talking her through the valley of the shadow of death.

Tessie's words and prayers allow Ruth to relax, and blood begins to flow. When the blood is drawn, glimmers of Ruth's vibrant personality show and she says, "I like all this attention."

I don't believe that Tessie has the power to make Ruth's body follow her pleas for healing. Imagery helps Ruth have some sense of control. It at least helps her to sleep more peacefully. Who understands the mind's power over the body; who is to say help can't come from this simple yet very resourceful method? Not me. At least it lets Ruth feel she has some power over her own health.

Later in the day Tessie speaks softy using the idea of warm sand, flowing water, and the beach as imagery. With her eyes, she motions me to take over. Tessie's voice is exhausted.

I freeze. Suddenly my mind is fused with color. All I can see is bright red, strong yellow. I shake my head. No! I can't speak. I try to tell Tessie. Color! Red! Yellow! My eyes can only see red, strong lines of red and clear yellow patterns. What? What? What does the color red and the color yellow mean? Embarrassed. Confused. I downplay the vision. Later when I can speak I tell Tessie, "Maybe the bright color means someday in the future Ruth will be well and sit on a beach in a yellow bathing suit under a bright red umbrella."

I cannot bring myself to tell Tessie how strong the image has affected me, so I foolishly tease, "I can't help it. Maybe even in these terrible moments my thoughts are too colorful for the quiet art of imaging." I have no way to know there is another meaning. Is it Ruth's red blood? Is it her sickly yellow skin? Someday the very words *red* and *yellow* will trigger the memory of this moment. Red. Yellow. It will alter everything I believe.

During this horrendous period, Ruth's physicians have reached an end to their medical ability to save her. It feels like they've begun withdrawing emotionally. Ruth is furious. Detachment is a device physicians often call upon to help distance emotions. Sometimes they come six or more at a time into the room. Today they enter Ruth's room, stand in a semicircle holding their books close to their bodies. No one introduces anyone. Ruth hates this cold impersonal approach. She tells them so without taking away their dignity. "It is disturbing to be this ill and have physicians whose names are not even given to you. I don't know your name or your name." She points to each one standing in the semi-circle. Each doctor immediately gives his or her first name.

Paul takes comfort from Ruth's words. "She gave them an eloquent, impassioned appeal to treat her with aggressive medicine, but asked them not to take her hope away by their suddenly withdrawing now that she has developed graft-versus-host disease."

Tessie tells Ruth, "You are still ministering here from your bed in the hospital. The lesson you have given those doctors will serve to help many patients as long as those physicians practice medicine."

Saturday morning Ruth seems so much better. We feel good enough about her condition to make plans to return home. She doesn't ask us to stay. "So, you think I am going to live?" she light-heartedly asks.

Sugarbaker says, "We do, or we wouldn't leave you."

Ruth acknowledges by saying, "That makes sense." She looks at me intently and says, "You, you will come back?"

"Tell Robin to call me if you need me, and I'll come back immediately," I respond.

On Sunday, we are back in Jackson. I feel a great need to be in my church. I feel safer about Ruth but afraid and tired and full of emotion about what it is like to see someone you love existing on a fine line between life and death.

Two lines from the Scripture catch my eye.

. . .if you continue in your faith, established and firm, not moving from the hope held out in the Gospel . . .

And then the lines,

. . .To this end I labor, struggling with all His energy, which so powerfully works in me . . .

When I read the "Time of Response," it says:

. . .As we go from here today, may we have the gifts of: the compassion and resourcefulness of the Good Samaritan, the energy of Martha, and the inner peace of Mary. And may we have the wisdom to know when to call upon each of these gifts.

I find myself smiling. Whatever Ruth needed from us in these terrible days she received as best we knew how to give. Compassion, energy, inner peace, and, yes, even curiosity were present. Each one of us brought to Ruth's room what was needed at the moment. All we can do is wait and pray.

Oh God

Why
Sit on a fence
Condemning
Simplistic things

Those folks who believe
God's parking
Appears at the perfect moment
With prayer

It's OK
Some need to believe
You'd care
Who parks where

Do
You
Answer prayer?

Is it enough to know You are there?
You have your own way with people who pray.

I walk and breathe
Prayer
Some days you must laugh to hear me say
I don't know you.

Amen.

Elizabeth

Chapter Nine

Fill My Cup, Lord

This, in a nutshell, is that will: that everything handed over to me by the Father be completed—not a single detail missed—and at the wrap-up of time I have everything and everyone put together, upright and whole. This is what my Father wants: that anyone who sees the Son and trusts who he is and what he does and then aligns with him will enter real life, eternal life. My part is to put them on their feet alive and whole at the completion of time. (John 6:39, from The Message *by Eugene Peterson)*

Tuesday after we return, the senior minister at church calls. "Ruth is dying," he pauses, his voice wobbles. "She wants to come back to Mississippi."

I hang up the telephone and sit down staring out the window at my backyard. I learned how to be happy long ago. *Have someone you can love. Have something you love doing.* Right now all I can muster from these truths about happiness is insufficient. Doesn't a person who can love even the lowest of flowers deserve happiness? I count on my flowers for solace. I planted them in the earth. I can smell them, see them, touch their petals, and hold them close. They're real; they exist. Do you, God? Are you really here with me when I'm faded? Wilting? Dying of thirst? Fill my cup, Lord. I'm just an empty old vase with a large crack so subtle it doesn't show until the flowers are carefully arranged. It's too late when the breath of life seeps out in small puddles. A little bit of glue just won't do, Lord. It's not enough.

Ruth's going to die and I hurt like when mother died. I was a five-year-old. It's as bad as it was when I said goodbye to Dad when he died. I was a young bride. The anguish brings back all the pain of having lost so much love. It tumbles in. So many close friends have died over the years. The faces of children with cancer with whom I've done volunteer work over the last twenty-five years flash before me. A distressing, somber parade of dead children. Right now I can't even recall all the children I also knew who lived. Ruth's going to die, and that knowledge brings all my questions of God to the forefront.

"No, God," I angrily say out loud, "this is too much loss." I wish now that I had not let myself love Ruth. "God, why do you let me love so much? I wish now I didn't know how to love." Deep anger and hurt for Ruth and her family grip my spirit. I can hardly bear the idea that Ruth has much left she wants to do, so many important plans for her life. Death will take her away, unfinished in this world.

Even in the midst of the worst of this reverie, there is one thought that overshadows the intense pain. I cannot resist worrying that when I see Ruth once again she will ask me if I think she is dying. I would rather face anything but those intense blue eyes watching me try to answer. Only days ago I told Ruth, "I have a great sense of life when I am near you. I think you are going to live." The words echo in my head. No human can grant power to keep someone alive. I know that, but even so, I feel I've let go of a thread of strong hope for life. Now that frail thread is broken, severed. There is the devastating possibility she will ask me this question again. I cannot bear to look into Ruth's eyes and answer, "You are dying."

Over in Atlanta, Sarah, one of Ruth's minister friends from seminary days, is staying at the hospital as arrangements to fly Ruth back to Mississippi are completed. Sarah calls and says, "Ruth has been hallucinating all day. She went into the bathroom and told us, 'I am not coming out until Jesus tells me to come out.' Ruth's mind has been racing. Her voice is filled with desperation. She's been giving intense instructions. Odd statements, all day," Sarah whispers in to the telephone.

At the end of this long, terrible day, Sarah goes into the room where Ruth is and tells her, "I need to tell you goodbye. I must go back to Birmingham."

Ruth suddenly becomes very still. She speaks clearly for the first time in many hours. "Sarah," Ruth says, "I have so much to tell you. There is more! So much more! More even than we knew!"

Shocked, Sarah realizes Ruth has told her something very important. I don't know what I believe about Ruth's words. Do people that near death come so close to whatever follows while at the same moment they still live and breathe in this world? Sarah and Ruth chose long ago to become ordained ministers in the Baptist church. It has been a difficult struggle here in the Deep South, but they reached their goal. Ruth's words confirm for Sarah her belief that God is real. She feels that Ruth, so close to death, has reached some level of communication that we, too fully living, know nothing about. Could it be possible? I've always known in death there is a presence, an unmistakable presence. Little children with cancer know it. I've felt it clearly when in their hospital rooms. In death it seems we are not alone. No other time do I feel such strength of presence. In death and dying there is no way to deny God seems very real. There can be little doubt that Ruth, the Ruth who has always believed in God, may very well have become privy to sacred knowledge. "There is more," she told Sarah. "So much more! More even than we knew."

Later Sarah tells me, "Ruth is determined to come back to Mississippi. She wants to be with her friends and family now." Then she adds, "I believe she spent today talking to God."

I can't help wondering if Ruth asked Him if He would let her stay alive long enough to come home to all of us one last time. My belief is that the Ruth I know well is still not ready to give up on living. She believes in God, has great faith. She is not afraid of what comes after life. I had asked her during this hard summer, "Ruth, what do you believe about life after death?"

She told me, "I believe. Heaven may not be just the way we think it will be. It may be different from our concept of heaven, but I know that this life is not the end of things. God is real. He has greater plans for us. I know it."

Now she's coming home to die, but I know Ruth is not finished living. She hopes that when she gets back to Mississippi the doctor who diagnosed her illness will be able to save her life. He has spoken as a friend to her, encouraged her to come back home. "I will take care of you," he has told Ruth. Later, when Ruth gets back to Mississippi, he will have to speak as her physician.

The Emory doctors have done all they can do for Ruth. Now, it seems they are not entering her room these last two days. Ruth and Robin feel deeply hurt by this unforgivable apparent abandonment. Only the one physician, the kind one who befriended Ruth from the beginning, comes into her hospital room at this stage of her transplant. Even he comes into the room only one time.

Each time I phone them, her sister whispers with great distress in her voice, "Ruth is so hurt and saddened by the doctors. We feel they have deserted us. We're alone."

Ruth chose these doctors to do the marrow transplant. They promised to do their best for her. She's been the center of their attention for fifty days and nights. I am incensed that now when they realize she is dying, they've mentally moved on to the next patient. Do they teach doctors that their jobs do not end when the patient is dying? Some doctors, fully human, seem to be at a loss about how to behave when a patient is dying. Others, such as the doctors I've seen working with childhood cancer, stay involved with their patients even if they are dying. There is no sense of desertion.

This feeling of desertion is something I felt early in my life. Forsaken. Rage at the idea that Ruth is feeling alone fuels flickering flames within my soul. The tears I weep cannot smother the raging fire deep inside of me. I give in to overwhelming grief and weep tears that will not subside.

In the eighteen hours before Ruth returns to Mississippi, our church prepares a home for her. We take her furniture out of storage and paint Ruth's new bedroom soft blue, the color she requests. We get a new home ready for her last homecoming in less than a day. Everyone works round-the-clock. It gives each person something to do for Ruth. It's important to surround her with her own belongings, however brief this time.

Placing a call to her hospital room, I tell Robin, "Sugarbaker and Tessie found a great condo for Ruth. Everyone from the church is waiting for her return to Mississippi. We'll be standing there when the plane lands with our arms opened wide. We will hold you both. We love you. We will never abandon you!"

As we wait, word from the hospital keeps getting worse. Sarah calls saying, "Ruth is deteriorating so rapidly that her skin is turning black."

Sugarbaker asks at some point during those terrible hours of waiting for Ruth's return, "What if she dies before she gets home? She will never see the beautiful home we have prepared for her."

"It will not be important," I tell her. "The only thing that matters now is that for one whole day Ruth has known that we prepared a place for her."

All that day Ruth tells Robin and anyone who comes into the room, "They're painting my new bedroom. I'll have a new home waiting for me. These people can move mountains."

God

Where are you?

With Ruth?

With Me?

Do
You
Hear me?

Forget:
Mansions in the sky
Streets of gold

Pearly white gates
St. Peter's trumpet, too

Ruth's earthly home will do

We've
Prepared it

Painted
Furnished
With
Love.

Is
Life
Sacrifice

Sufficient
Unto you?

Amen.

You know it's me,
Elizabeth

Chapter Ten

I Remember My Promise

Tessie, Sugarbaker, and I understand on one level that Ruth is coming home to die; even that she may not live long enough to get home. But it is only after the plane lands at the airfield with Ruth aboard that I feel myself truly accepting that our sweet friend cannot live in this condition. The door to the airplane opens. We see her bright smile and hear her words, "I am home!"

I move though heavy, clouded water, slowing my breath, echoing my heartbeat. I know I can do whatever I must, but the enormous effort causes terrible pain as I adjust to the fact that our friend is locked inside a body that no longer has the strength to live in this world.

Ruth's words spoken to me when she had first been diagnosed vibrate in my mind: *"I am going to lean hard on you. My family will not be able to bear that I have cancer. You are one of the few people I know who can handle something like this."*

I remember my promise. *"I am strong and I will help you do whatever you must do."*

Yesterday, I promised Ruth and her sister, " I will not abandon you."

Tessie, Sugarbaker, and I stand close together, bracing each other. Sugarbaker shouts, "Yeh! Hurrah!"

Tessie and I join in, "Yeh! Hurrah, you're home."

Sugarbaker and I step toward Ruth. Tessie and our Senior Minister stand back. Their faces reflect shock and pain at Ruth's condition. Only Sugarbaker and I move forward and begin talking to Ruth. Our voices disguise broken hearts.

Ruth says, "I saw two rainbows on the way home."

"We arranged them for you," I say, so frightened by the reality of her condition that I can't stay silent.

Ruth is happy to be home; she's glad to see us. Her big eyes shine. It's hard to see how she could be alive in such a frail body. "Y'all, I promise you, there was a shadow on one of the rainbows. It was in the exact shape of the state of Mississippi," she says. We laugh. Ruth is always full of surprises.

Ruth is then carefully loaded into the waiting ambulance. We put cool cloths on her forehead. Rub ice on her arms. Adjust to the reality. Our dear Ruth is locked inside this destroyed shell of a body. Fifty-five days ago she had not even looked ill.

Later, after Ruth is settled into her new home, she looks at me and says out of the blue, "You. You are centered."

I ask Ruth, "Did you mean self-centered?"

"No, I said you are a centered person."

Confused, I nod my head and smile at Ruth. It will take me a while to understand what she has told me.

Later I tell her mother Maude about Ruth seeing the rainbow shadow. Maude smiles and says, "Now, she knows good and well that was only the state of Tennessee turned backwards."

Maude and Robin don't seem to accept that Ruth is dying. But we have been told Ruth will go into a coma soon, and then she will die. We have no way of knowing the day. Soon. She has one week left to live. We only know we want to be here with her. We want to help her live every moment of whatever time she has left in this world. We surround Ruth with her own earthly belongings she has missed so much in the stark hospital. We show her love in every human manner as we helplessly wait for her death.

After everyone leaves the condo, I settle down on Ruth's sofa for a sleepless night. I remember the words the ambulance driver told Tessie. "If one of you has to call for an ambulance, remember we are legally bound to resuscitate Ruth if you don't have a paper from the doctor saying otherwise." I pull Paul aside and explain.

"Please call the doctor and take care of getting the paper from him," he tells me.

As much as we want Ruth to live, her body is too ill to do so. We can't hold her where she is not physically able to belong.

God

Reverend Ruth says
I'm centered.
I asked,
Did you mean
Self-centered?
No, she said,
You are centered.

My daughter-in-law says I am flamboyant.
My friends say I am funny and fun.
My landscape customers say
"You are talented and so organized."

I say
Thank you
Out loud

And
Think to myself

Oh, My Gosh,
I hope I haven't locked my keys in the car.

Who am I?
Help me love the real me.

Amen.

Elizabeth

Chapter Eleven

Dealing with Angels

After Ruth is resting for the night, Maude says, "You don't have to leave, do you? Can't you stay tonight?" My husband is out of town tonight, so it is fine with me to stay. Later, I fall into a light sleep on the sofa, and Robert, Ruth's longtime friend who's come from Florida to be with Ruth, wakes me.

"Ruth's legs are hurting. Paul wants to know if we can warm some towels to put on her legs." We wet the towels; the microwave doesn't work so I stand ironing them hot. For hours Robert runs a relay of fresh hot towels back and forth to Ruth's room. I'm so relieved to actually be doing something helpful for Ruth that I don't get tired.

The afternoon of the next day I go home and sleep for a while. It's a shock when I return. Sugarbaker and Tessie have located a wheelchair and Ruth is using all her energy and willpower to take a look at her condo. I am so encouraged! I sit down on the sofa and think maybe she can live. Ruth points to her bald head. "Give me a kiss," she says. I find myself unable to move, unable to give that hello kiss.

"No, Ruth I'm too hot and sticky. I'm afraid I'll give you something." Ruth points to the top of her head once again. But I can't move. I'm thinking, *she's dying; no, maybe she's going to live.* Ruth had looked in every room of the condo. Some of the things in the condo are not Ruth's own belongings. Church friends helped get the rooms ready and added things to make it prettier. Ruth asks me, "Can we give back the things that aren't mine?"

Confused, I am horrified to hear myself asking her, "Do you mean afterwards?" I stumble, recover and say, "Sure, I'll take care of it."

Later Robert and I talk. He says, "Ruth has a great need to be surrounded by nothing but her own familiar belongings. She's been lonely not only for her friends, but also for the things that she connected with her happy life."

We have no way to know if she even has one week left to live. The doctors have warned us it will be only days. I mentally divide up this precious time. The first night I call "Show Time," but after that first night I accept we're in "Real Time." There is no way of knowing how long it would be until Ruth goes from being very aware to entering a state of coma. *Get it in your head,* I tell myself. *Ruth's dying.*

Tonight while everyone sleeps I change the setting of the condo into a place that requires less energy and less stimulation. For the first time in my life, flowers give me no pleasure. The mums that seemed so lovely on "Show Time" are too bright and far too gay to be inside. Outside they go. Anything that is not familiar to Ruth I put away. Ruth needs all her strength to live through days so painfully numbered. Ruth loves angels. One church friend has placed many angels from Ruth's collection around the house and added some of her own.

Robert comments, "Ruth likes angels, but soon they are going to be her new neighbors. She does not want to deal with them right now." I put the angels into the closet.

The next day I tell Ruth, "There is nothing in your new home except the things you most love and that belong to you. Now, this house looks more like people who don't really know how to decorate, like you and me." She smiles.

Ruth's bedroom is cool with a wall of glass that lets her see out into the green trees outside her window. We remove the hospital bed and put her in her own brass bed.

Robin and Paul spend twenty-four hours a day in the room with Ruth, taking care of her needs. Throughout the nights, Robin's two sons and Paul's daughter slip into the room and kiss their beloved

Aunt Ruth. All of Ruth's family is here staying in the condo as Ruth clings to life.

"I can live here as long as I want to," she tells us. Is Ruth pretending she's not dying because she wants to give her family time to be better prepared for her death? Could it be for our sakes? The question haunts me. Does Ruth still believe that she will live? There is much hugging and holding among her friends and family. We are locked into loving Ruth toward her death.

When I sit by Ruth's bedside I remember for some strange reason the words from some of Ruth's and my favorite hymns. Songs, the-take-me-back-to-my-roots hymns, not commonly sung in churches like North Baptist. "'Tis So Sweet to Trust in Jesus." "Count Your Blessings, Name Them One by One." "Precious Lord, Take My Hand." Songs from Ruth's childhood and my own.

I sit here, words echoing in my head. Watching Ruth die. I feel disbelief. How can someone once so full of life be dying? I feel numb. It's the only way I can bear more pain. I feel disbelief again. How could someone so full of life be dying?

I feel full of love. Overflowing love. For Ruth. For her precious family. For our church family as they meet Ruth's every need.

I feel God's presence. I question Him but can't be near Ruth and continually question God. He is in this house. He is in Ruth's fragile face.

He has always been in the rooms of children with cancer for whom I've done so much volunteer work over the years. The dying children often recognize Him. I could always see it clearly. Now He is here with Ruth and her family. Why do I have so much trouble fully believing in God? Maybe God brings the love that surrounds Ruth. We could bear such loss no other way.

Maude, not understanding the damage of liver failure, often says, "Look how they have burned my Ruth's body with radiation." The tenderhearted men from the church who come every day to help lift Ruth pale when they see her. Everyone helps in some way. The best cooks in the church prepare every meal. When all the peach pie is gone, Maude wonders aloud, "Wonder if Mabel plans to bake us another one?"

"Your new peach pie will be here tomorrow," I tell Maude after making a phone call to the church.

Maude frowns and teases, "I guess that means we will have to go the whole night without it." We laugh through broken hearts, and it helps soften the pain.

The children of the church are still praying for a miracle that will save Ruth's life. Can prayer alter the course of Ruth's life? How will the children handle it when they don't get their miracle?

Sugarbaker's child, twelve-year-old Courtney, adores Ruth. "Courtney is the child who should have been born to me," Ruth always says.

Today Courtney brings a dream chaser to Ruth and tells her, "The breeze blows the feathers and chases bad dreams away and brings good dreams."

Ruth tells her, "I want the good dreams."

Courtney is waiting for a miracle. She believes Ruth will live. Sugarbaker has struggled to help young Courtney prepare for Ruth's death. But Courtney clings to the belief that if you pray hard enough and often enough, God will intervene. Today Courtney lies down beside her dear Ms. Ruth on her deathbed. I watch Courtney holding Ruth's hand. Courtney plays with Ruth's little dog, Cleo. Courtney kisses Cleo, and then kisses Ruth.

Ruth sleeps after a while. I silently pray, don't let this experience leave Courtney scarred for life.

"Can you sleep for a while, Courtney?"

Courtney nods. I hand her a pillow. She closes her eyes. Ruth's head slips to one side. Before I can move Courtney sits up, gently straightens Ruth's head and gives Ruth more kisses. Courtney doesn't see Ruth's damaged body. She sees only the beloved personage of her Ms. Ruth.

Courtney expects a miracle.

There are moments when we all have hope. It's so hard to believe that God would let Ruth die.

I don't believe God sends what we interpret as miracles. I have watched too many parents beg God for healing for children dying with cancer. I've never seen it happen. But I find myself relishing the miracles that surround Ruth: her passion for life, her utter belief in God. Leukemia and disappointment have not changed her faith. Even in the process of detaching from this earth, Ruth doesn't lose the miracle of joy. Dying doesn't change the beauty of Ruth's human spirit. Nor does she lose her love for music and laughter.

Ruth tries to make sure that we help each other endure her dying. She articulates to each of us the value she sees within our own selves.

"You," she told me, "are a centered person."

To Robin, her sister, Ruth says, " You have so much kindness in you. What would I have done without you?"

To her brother Paul she says, "You are such a fine man, such a good brother. I have always known I could depend on you."

Late in the evening a friend from church stops by to see Ruth. "Oh, how pretty!" Ruth says when she sees her friend's necklace.

"I got it in Israel. You can keep the necklace for a while if you would like." Nora Jane hangs the necklace of gold with a tiny jug of holy water from Israel on Ruth's brass bed.

Later in the night Robert and Paul lift Ruth beside her bed so that Robin can change her gown. They lose their balance. Fall. Break the frame of Ruth's bed. "Ruth's going to kill us if she realizes the mess we've made of her brass bed," Robert says.

The bed tilts over at a sharp angle. Nora Jane's beautiful necklace is crushed. Shocked, I watch the holy water flow across Ruth's pillows, anointing Ruth's bed in an unexpected but appropriate blessing.

Ruth is too ill too notice the condition of her bed. She deteriorates more each day. I don't know which is worse—having Ruth so clear-headed and desperately ill or watching her body shut down more and more.

Hymns and Bible phrases from my childhood float into my head from my subconscious. "Blessed Assurance." "If It Were Not So, I Would Not Have Told You." "Love Lifted Me." The messages are clear. These old familiar words provide comfort and guidance as I fight to live through terrible hours of loss.

Watching. Waiting. Knowing. Ruth's dying.

Lord

I owe you

The
Miracle
Of
Unexpected
Anointment

Holiness
In the middle
Of
Pain

Solace

Children
Who
Kiss
Sorrow

Words that float;
Blessed Assurance. Love Lifted Me.

Heal
My doubt.

Amen.

Elizabeth

Chapter Twelve

Independently Dependent

Each person is given a job that they are best able to perform during the last few days of Ruth's life. Mine seems to be to help Maude live through this terrible time. The more self-assured and in-charge Tessie and Sugarbaker become, the more I step back and let them do the busy work, bathe Ruth, keep up with medical reports, make decisions. Ruth's condition unnerves me so I can't follow simple direction from Tessie and Sugarbaker on how to fold a blanket Ruth needs placed under her legs. I know I'm meant to be here. I promised Ruth I would not leave her. Sometimes I'm just so scared. I have this idea of who I am. It took a long time to become self-confident, sure of myself. I'm losing self-confidence. But this morning Maude defines the way she sees the three of us by saying, "There is our sweet Sugarbaker. Tessie is the one filled with the Holy Spirit, but when we need heart, it is you that we need."

It takes all three of us and a whole church of friends to meet the needs of Ruth's family. To Robin and Paul we are almost the same as one person.

Not one of us has any way to know where we fit in Ruth's life before she was ill. Only Ruth knows and now she is too ill for it to matter.

"Let's visit," she used to tell me.

"Do you want to talk, or do you want me to talk?" I would ask.

Sometimes we'd have what Ruth called "kissie" talk. I knew that, as a single gal, she loved to hear about such things. "I'll draw on my sister's love life today," I once told her. "As an old married woman, my love life is too ordinary to be interesting."

"I get so tired of happily married folks trying to convince me that I'm not missing anything," Ruth had replied.

"My single sister is in love," I'd told Ruth. "When my other sister told her how pretty she's looking, she responded by saying, 'You'd look good, too, if you had spent the morning floating around in a swimming pool with someone kissing on your toes!'"

Ruth had laughed at the image this little story gave her. "Oh, how funny," she said.

If I get too still or alone I find myself replaying conversations Ruth and I had after she was diagnosed with cancer. Sometimes Ruth would tease, "I'm going to be so mad at Jesus if I die before I've ever had sex."

The most difficult part of Ruth's dying is that the unfairness of an early death will leave Ruth with so much living left undone. She wanted to have children. She had so much to give to the world—so many spirit-filled gifts to share.

How can we bear what Ruth must bear? Why would a just God be so unjust?

Can you pray a person well? Can enough folks pray so long and so truly that God will hear them and answer their prayers? Are prayers just empty words, bouncing off walls with no ceilings?

Prayer brings the blessing of strength, making it possible to live through whatever you must bear. Prayer can bring peace; it can bring serenity. Can it change or alter the course of death? I don't think so, but sometimes prayers seem to be answered in unexpected moments.

Chapter Thirteen

Help Coming from the Lord

Help coming from the Lord? Help in the form of a friend comes to Ruth's front door. A member of our church stops by to help lift Ruth and brings his guitar with him.

Ruth's brother asks, "Would you like to sing for Ruth?"

"I would be honored."

Some of us sit on the floor, some on the edge of the extra bed, and others stand; we surround Ruth's bed, filling the small room. The music begins and the singing starts. There are those who have clear beautiful voices. Others like me wobble, crack, and stammer, but we all sing.

"Breathe on me, breath of God . . ."

Ruth, propped by five large pillows, lies in her own brass bed. The edges of her eyelids are ulcerated, red, raw, and protruding beyond intense deep blue eyes. The liver failure distorts her swollen face. Her blotched skin is a sickly mustard with dark blue splotches. And yet, she is singing quietly with a muted energy that needs to be a part of the world she loves.

"Great is thy faithfulness!"

We sing until our throats become parched. I ask for water, move around the room, gently handing each friend a cup. *"Take this, drink, in the name of God the Father,"* I hear inside my head. Mysterious words? Perhaps! I look into the faces in this room and see pure affection combined with raw pain as we take part in a communion of fellowship and love. Only music can satisfy my need to express the powerful emotions I am experiencing.

"Thou art the bread of life, O send thy spirit, Lord, now unto me."

We surround Ruth's bed, our voices exploding with song. I shed my shield of protective armor that warns "don't feel." Ruth's truth—that she's dying—deserves more. I open myself, unguarded, and experience a force more powerful than a mere frail world. Unmistakably, a Presence lifts us upward as we sing.

"I come to the garden alone, while the dew is still on the roses"

I am the soloist. Ruth knows I sing my favorite song, my soft, shaken voice now firm, blatant, blazing.

"And He walks with me, and He talks with me"

Does someone walk with me, counsel me? I know death stalks our friend; *he* is in this room. Is some other presence also here? Then let Ruth live!

Maude seems almost peaceful in these moments of singing. She leans near to the bed, patting her child's arms. These songs have immeasurable meaning to them both, and I watch in wonder as mother and daughter transmit a lifetime of shared faith. Then, we sing what Maude says is her favorite hymn.

"How firm a foundation, ye saints of the Lord . . . I am with thee. O be not dismayed."

The galloping plunge of painful reality approaching, our golden friend's deathbed becomes more than I can bear. Grief overcomes the joy of singing. I weep, tremble, and silently seek peace. Singing words that my shallow pride cannot speak, I lay my head against the shoulder of our young minister, Stan.

"I am weak, but Thou art strong . . ."

The guitarist lays the instrument across his legs and asks Ruth, "How would you like for us to sing some Christmas songs next?"

"Oh yes, let's do," she says with a surprising energetic smile.

I think, *oh, no, the Christmas songs!* Ruth loves Christmas. This will be the last time she ever gets to hear the Christmas songs. "Yes, yes," I murmur, "of course we must sing them."

The penetrating heat of August blisters the windows lining the bedroom wall, sapping strength away. But here in Ruth's room, the air is cool as we stand around her deathbed singing. The sunlight is fading. The wind shakes green trees growing beside the window, forcing them to bow down. Green limbs, wavy wings, brush against plate glass. I sit on the edge of the bed and listen to the sound of mighty force. The trees stagger; their roots burrow deep. They cling like Ruth and me to earth. I close my eyes and humbly bow my own head. The light is going out. Darkness is falling. We sing:

"Silent night, holy night . . ."

Ruth closes exhausted eyes and drifts to sleep. Her tense body uncoils.

Beliefs transcend death, the hymns remind me. Tonight when I lie down on the sofa, I give up questioning and fall into deep sleep.

The next afternoon a different group of Ruth's friends comes by to sing for her and put together a spectacular floor show entertaining Ruth. We laugh with joy to see a glimpse of the Ruth we all knew before illness took its toll. "I like all this attention!" she laughs.

It is the last shimmering sparkle of her mischievous joy.

Ruth makes one request. "Let's sing 'I Surrender All'." This song ends denial. She sings with an acceptance given by a power beyond that of human strength.

"All to Him I freely give. I surrender all, all to Thee, my blessed Savior . . . All to Jesus I surrender, Lord, I give myself to Thee."

We sing and watch Ruth give in to death, a natural process at an unnatural time. Ruth's too young to die. She closes tired, accepting eyes and drifts into a deep sleep, which is the coma that we've feared.

The next day the coma continues to deepen. Her family spends the night singing for Ruth TV commercials and theme songs from television shows like *The Waltons* and *Gilligan's Island*. These, too, are a part of the life Ruth has loved. *The Partridge Family* theme song echos familiar words, "I think I looove you." Then, they sing the children's songs that Ruth loved as a child.

"The B-I-B-L-E, yes that's the book for me."

"Preacher, can I sing a song?" Ruth had asked as a small child long ago going down for her birthday pennies.

It is that song the family sings next.

"Let others see Jesus in you . . ."

Maude, eyes flooded with tears, joins in the harmony. Even in deep coma, Ruth faintly hums these sweet songs that call to her from childhood.

The peacefulness I've begun to claim drains away as I watch Ruth slipping deeper and deeper into coma, faintly alive. Inaudible gasping. Flesh dying. Ruth suddenly cries out, "Mommy, Mommy. Hurry Robin, hurry Robin!"

Maude tells me, "I believe her thoughts are going back into the past, as far back as the time when she was still my little girl, following along after me, calling to her sister, 'Hurry, hurry.'"

"Yes," I murmur and whimper inside my head the very words I've most wanted not to utter. "It is time now. Come, Lord. Take Ruth home."

Hurry, hurry.

Lord

Help me

Take my doubt

Praise words that sing
In
Silence and sadness.

Hold us in your strong hands

Amen.

Elizabeth

Chapter Fourteen

Absolute Tenderness

The next morning when I arrive back at Ruth's condo, Maude greets me saying, "I was a-wondering where you was."

"You OK, Maude?"

"Oh, I guess, for an old gal. That's my child a-laying in there. Everybody loves Ruth, but it's hardest on me."

"It must be terrible for you, Maude," I say. In a few moments we go into the kitchen and I say, "Come on, let me fix some breakfast for you."

Just as the eggs begin to fry, Paul walks into the kitchen. "Ruth has been throwing up blood. I think she will soon die."

I reach out and gently touch his arm. "Oh, Paul," I say. He manages a small smile, and goes straight back to Ruth's room.

I grab Maude in my arms. We have known that Ruth would die, but still we're not ready to let her go. Maude is still not prepared for Ruth's death. I say, "In the night I couldn't sleep thinking that we may need to let Ruth know that it is okay for her to let go. Would it be all right if I read to you what I have written down for Ruth?"

"Yes, I'd like to hear it," says Maude, and she sits down.

I read the words that I want to say to Ruth: "Do you feel well enough to listen to me right now? When we talked about my sense that you would have life and all the promises that it implied, I was thinking of life as I know it—life here on earth. The phrase 'Life Everlasting' keeps coming into my mind. Life Everlasting, a kind of life that I know nothing about. Do you think that it is possible? Life Everlasting, I mean? I bet you know so much more about that than I do right now. I realize that you may need to know that if you want to follow a different kind of life than what we talked about, your family can bear it now. You have helped them get to that place through your suffering. We'd miss you so much. If you decide to go before us, will you find all the good places to have fun and will you wait for us there? We love you and we'll miss you so much. And Ruth, thank you for all the hugs and the 'Hey, Honeys.' I love you so much."

Maude cries. Paul comes back into the breakfast room and asks me to call the hospice nurse. "Find out what we should prepare for now that Ruth is throwing up blood. Ask her what could happen that we may not know how to handle."

I lift the telephone, my hands shaking, but my voice is firm as I tell the hospice nurse what's happening and ask her questions that Paul needs answered.

"She may die quietly or she may lose a large volume of blood at death," the hospice nurse says. "Death should be within hours."

Paul and I sit down in the dining room together and I tell him what the nurse has said. When he has a moment to compose himself I say, "Paul, we called her doctor, too, and he said there are three ways we can handle things when Ruth dies. We can call an ambulance; we can call the funeral home; or we can call him and he will come by in a few hours after her death and take care of things."

"No ambulance," Paul answers.

I'm glad. The sound of a siren and the appearance of an ambulance would only add more pain.

"If we call the funeral home," Paul says, "I will not let anyone handle her body unless they have lost a mother or a sister. Whoever handles Ruth's body must use absolute tenderness."

"Yes," I say. "Yes. With tenderness." Ruth deserves it. Absolute tenderness!

"Will you call and tell the church?" Paul asks. "I think we should not have the volunteers in today."

"I'll call the church and send that word and then I'll go, too."

"No, please stay," he says. "We need you . . . you, Tessie, and Sugarbaker always can come and go and the ministers, too, of course. Will you keep Mama occupied?"

"You know I will."

Later, our senior minister comes to the house and I tell him what's been happening.

"Maybe we should gather more towels in case there is a lot of blood," he says.

I try to make a fresh pot of coffee. My pastor sees my hands shaking. He takes the coffeepot and says, "Let me make it." I nod and one cry escapes my lips. He wraps his arms around me and we stand one brief moment, both of us, shaken by our sadness.

I sit down at the table and hold a small silver frame that had been given to Ruth. Framed are the words, "Lo, though I walk through the valley of the shadow of death, I will fear no evil." My fingers trace the silver frame as I read the words over and over, trying to calm my body and come to grips with what this day will bring.

Today, with the family choosing to be alone with only those people whom they've come to know so well, it's strange as I send the helpers from the church away at the door, explaining the family's wishes.

In the afternoon Maude and I sit quietly in the living room. Some of the time we talk or fall into a fretful sleep. From time to time we look at the kitchen table and see the dirty dishes left from early morning. "We really should clean up the kitchen," we say. Then, we look at one another and ask, "Who really gives a hoot about the dishes?" The early morning image of Ruth throwing up blood and what that means leaves us in such painful knowledge that we sit on the sofa with our feet up in a chair and our hearts covered in sadness.

Later on, when we finally clean the kitchen, Maude grins and says, "Lordy, I sure hope we pass Tessie's kitchen inspection."

When Sugarbaker is free to drop by at the end of this day, I'm so exhausted I know I must go home and sleep for a while. I sleep for a few hours and then wake up so upset I literally chant out loud my pain. I pour out my grief and try to hold on to my sanity. I lament, "Come by here Lord, Come by here Lord. It is time for the Amen, Lord. It is time for the Amen, Lord." My prayers for Ruth's life have changed from a prayer for her life to a prayer for God to take the spirit of the person who's no longer present in her own body.

During the time I've spent with Ruth's family I could contain my emotions. Away from Ruth's house I lose it. In the night I take the theme from an old spiritual called "Kumbayah" as my lament to God.

Come by here.
Come and see what you've done.
Come by here.
Your little girl is almost done.
Come by here
Lift her up, Lord
Come by here.
Cure what you've done, Lord.
Help us to forgive what you've done.
With our eyes to the setting sun
I hate what you've done, Lord.
Take what you've done, Lord.
If we must be awake, Lord
Help us take what you've done.
Free our girl, Lord.
How will we live, Lord,
Without our girl.
Sometimes I must hate you, Lord.
See what you've done
Free our girl, Lord.
How proud you must be,
Lord, of your girl.
With our eyes to the setting sun

Now is the time for the Amen, Lord.
Thank you for your girl,

Thank you for your girl.
Amen, Amen, Amen.
Absolute tenderness, Lord.
Thank you, Lord!

I know Ruth's soul is longing to depart from this world. It's time to complete the covenant she made as a small child so many years ago. I cannot bear for Ruth to stay in a body that seems to be keeping her where she no longer belongs.

At two o'clock in the morning I drive over to Ruth's house. On the way, I remember the hospice nurse saying that when she dies, she could die quietly, or she could expel large volumes of blood. I can't bear for the family to have to deal with such a sight.

The door has been left unlocked, and I let myself inside. When I enter the house everyone is sleeping. I pick up a large stack of towels and spread one on the floor in the hall in front of Ruth's door and lie down. If the blood comes at Ruth's death I can be ready. The towels could conceal any blood. I gather my courage. Ruth sleeps in Paul's arms, resting peacefully.

So I rest, sometimes thinking, sometimes sleeping. Someday I will go see the mountain Ruth loves. I think about Maude who taught Ruth such wisdom. "Always remember, child, sin is like soot on snow," she had told her.

I want to know how a sister can love so deeply that she'd leave her children, give up her job security to stay with her beloved sister in a hospital room for fifty days and nights, loving and praying for a miracle? How will she feel when it doesn't arrive? How does a brother love so completely that even in the face of despair he leaves his job, brings his whole family to be with his sister in a place of her own choice? Ruth wanted to be here with her church family. How have we given them the love that they have needed? Ruth's every earthly need has been met. From where does that kind of love come? It must come from beyond our prideful, selfish selves.

The light gently rises outside the window as I lay on my towel bed. Early in the morning as the household wakes, Sugarbaker comes into the kitchen. We hug each other. While I lay sleeping on the floor near Ruth's door, Sugarbaker was sleeping just a few feet away in the next room in a sleeping bag. Neither of us knew the other was in the house. And so it is that the two of us are here when Ruth takes one deep breath, then another, smiles one last time, and dies in Paul's arms.

"Call Tessie, call Tessie," Maude tells us. Tessie is there in moments.

For more than a year we've prayed and begged on bended knee, "Let Ruth live her life."

Has it been only one week since Ruth asked me, "Elizabeth, do you think I am going to die?"

"I feel a great sense of life when I am near you," I'd told her.

When they take Ruth's body out of the condo, we walk solemnly behind the gurney. Her brother Paul, her sister Robin, Tessie, Sugarbaker, Ruth's friend Robert, and me. No one can bear to cover Ruth's sweet face. Sunlight suddenly casts a bright light across her body. Paul says, "We can cover Ruth's face now."

Tessie says, "I feel as though we should salute and that bugles should be blowing."

Absolute tenderness
God, Father, Son, and Holy Ghost
Saved
Our suffering
Ruth
Whose
Calm quiet smile
Greets and waves goodbye
Leaving
Unknown
Warriors
Surrendering
Golden Smile

This
Sad delight
How
Bitter sweet
Is
Thy guided wings' flight

Elizabeth

Chapter Fifteen

Ruth's Flowers

The morning after Ruth's death, I look outside at the many containers of flowers in my garden. All this sad summer, the sight of them has been one of the few things that seemed to offer comfort for the horrible feeling of fear for Ruth's life. A gentle rain is falling on the blossoms. The notion that God could be weeping upon the very flowers that He created strikes me as hopeful myth. I hope God does weep! Long bitter tears.

Only a few months ago the great hall at the church held the celebration party for Ruth's blessing of a bone marrow donation. Now it holds her body beneath a pall. The room, once filled with laughter and hope, holds our friend just this one last time. Friends greet Ruth's family and tell the many stories of how Ruth's faith and care enriched their lives and the lives of their children.

Robin and Paul minister to the children of our church on this terrible day. No miracle saved their beloved Ms. Ruth. Robin speaks, oh so gently, to the bewildered children. She bends down to one child and says, "Oh, Ms. Ruth told me about your beautiful eyes," and the little child replies with all the confidence Ms. Ruth had helped her to attain. "Uh-hm, and they turn different colors in the sunlight."

The children who have given Ruth such joy now deal with her death with poise. Ruth helped teach them that to love is a great and glorious thing. She gave them confidence. They know what it is to be loved by family and friends. Ruth showed them how to love.

One child is dressed in a long, flowing flower girl dress. She wears a tiara and her mother's rhinestones. She says, "I want to honor Ms. Ruth." Another child is wearing her tap shoes for much the same reason.

Earlier in the day I told Maude, "There will be so many flowers. Let me have your hair done for you instead of buying flowers for Ruth's funeral." Tonight she runs her fingers through her hair and says, "These are Ruth's flowers."

I couldn't resist buying one of those musical cards that caught my eye. I hand it to Maude and she tells me, "I just hope nothing jumps out at me!"

When she opens the card, many colorful birds jump out and the message reads, "All the birds in heaven are whistling at you."

The next morning we take Maude into the sanctuary to look at the funeral pall that will be used to cover Ruth's casket. A North Church friend quietly explains the meaning of each symbol done in beautiful blue and brick red threads of crewelwork. Organ music plays softly in the background as the church organist prepares for the funeral service to be held the next morning.

"The cross is a statement about the nature of God's love. It is the emblem of atonement and the symbol of salvation and redemption through Christianity," says the friend, pointing out the designs on the pall. "The intertwined ovals represent the Trinity—Father, Son, and Holy Spirit. Blue, the color of the sky, symbolizes heaven and heavenly love. It is also the color of truth because blue always appears in the sky after the clouds have disappeared, suggesting the unveiling of truth. These expressions clearly represent all of Ruth's strong beliefs."

Afterward, we walk with Maude down the church hall toward Ruth's office. Maude stops and speaks to Mr. Jefferson, our custodian. "Mr. Jefferson, I know how much Ruth cared about you. I just want you to know that tomorrow, I am taking Ruth home."

I walk back into the church sanctuary and sit on my favorite pew. The cross hangs high above the organ on a blank wall. I am horrified to realize that in the past when I looked at this cross I've often felt peace. Now when I look, shadows fall across the image of the body of Ruth hanging there, a yellow-skinned, blood-covered body of my own disbelief.

How can I sit
In the center
Of
Disbelief
And
Watch
Ruth
Suspended
On your cross
Exposed to the world
Oh, Lord
Is it
Me?
My own inadequacies,
Laid bare.
So high up there
On
The
Cross
Of confusion?

Amen.

Elizabeth

Chapter Sixteen

Explicit Direction

Make no mistake, Ruth did what most folks never do. She directed her own death, letting us know in no uncertain terms what she needed, when she needed it, and from whom she needed it. She left explicit directions for her funeral, too.

We seem to be following subconscious directions even in our choice of funeral clothes. I've chosen my funeral costume with care. Maude took one look at me the first time we met and asked, "Do you just go out and buy them loud colors that you wear?"

"No," I had laughed. "They send me a catalog marked 'Loud Colors' and I just pick the ones that seem the brightest." Ruth would expect me to play my part by wearing a dress more fitting for a party than a funeral.

Ruth told another friend, Joan, "Joan, you must weep the loudest at my funeral." Of course, we hadn't believed at the time that Ruth would really die. Joan seems to be doing her part. She's weeping for real.

The congregation fills the room. Many of Ruth's friends from other cities and other churches who had been a part of her life are here today. Seminary friends who now live in Atlanta have driven over for the funeral. She has maintained many close relationships. We call these friends of Ruth's "The Atlanta Women." They visited with Ruth and Robin many days while she was hospitalized. They are in their best black dresses wearing long pearl necklaces. "We just know Ruth would want us to wear our best pearls to her funeral," they tell us.

Tessie is wearing her navy dress. Ruth always told her, "You look so professional in that dress."

Sugarbaker has all the pallbearers organized and makes sure they have little flowers pinned on their shoulders. As we sit waiting for the service to begin, suddenly the sound of an airplane flying low to the church roof overwhelms us with sound. I fear the worst. What if Ruth made plans to have something dropped down right on top of our humbled heads?

Thank goodness it was just an unusual occurrence.

When the loud sound ceases, Tessie steps forward to walk down the aisle in her role as pallbearer and smiles. Just as she enters the sanctuary, the hook on her bra comes undone. *Well,* she thinks, *I knew you would pull one last trick on me.*

Ruth's family is seated up front. The ceremony begins and the drama gets to full force. We read from the Litany of Praise, "As for Mortals, their Days are like grass; they flourish like a flower of the field, for the wind passes over and it is gone. But steadfast love of the Lord is from Everlasting to Everlasting . . ."

Ministers who had been such an important part of Ruth's life participate in the service. Sarah stands and reads from *Ordination* by James A. Autry, the poem that was given to Ruth by her radiologist.

> . . . And now the old preachers come to lay their hands
> on a new kind of preacher,
> a preacher from the seminary
> a preacher who studied the Bible in Greek
> and Hebrew,
> who knew about religions they never heard of,
> who knew about computers
> and memory banks full of sermons
> and many other modern things.
> A new kind of preacher,
> And yet,
> A preacher who still would feel on her head
> The hands
> Like a commandment
> From all the preachers and deacons who ever were . . .

Our senior pastor speaks about Ruth, saying, "Sometimes I think it is her laugh that I shall miss the most. It healed and smoothed and gave perspective . . . at the core of her being was the joyful spring that coursed through her living. And she was clear; we were made clear as to the source of that spring. It was her faith. It was her love for God's word, both the written word and the Living Word, in which she lived and moved and had her very being . . . ."

Our dear heart, young Stan, the church's youngest minister, reads with ardent clarity from the Old Testament, "I have called thee by name; Thou art mine, for I am the Lord thy God."

Then, one of Ruth's former ministers speaks, and my thoughts of death are changed forever. "God, our Redeemer, is such a redeemer that He makes logic of even this or He has let us down hard. Are we justified in letting Him down as well? There is no middle ground. We have to choose."

He pauses and wipes his own tears. "I suspect Ruth was born for that very purpose. To stand and call people to make life's most important choices."

No! I think. *No! Why would God use Ruth's life only to take it when she wanted desperately to live?*

"God will be able to account for everything, including all that has happened to Ruth . . . *if He needs to.* But somehow, in that greater dimension of knowing, I really don't see us calling anybody to account for anything."

I shall! I angrily promise myself. *I need to know!*

Then the minister speaks the words that change my life. They take away my fear of death. "Somehow, in that greater dimension of knowing, I really don't see us calling anybody to account for anything. I suspect that all the issues of this life, all of the jubilant triumphs and all the devastating tragedies, so sharply focused and pertinent to us now, will fade fast when finally we meet the Lord. In the twinkling of an eye, the questions will be gone from our spiritual agenda. The follies and fallenness of man and mind and earth and body will, in the light of His glory and grace, be reduced to irrelevance. To persist in agonizing over former things will be worse than incongruous; it will be insensible, even laughable."

His words bring me full force into a new reality. If there is more after death, emotion will be related to life after death. Even emotions will be transformed. I feel stunned by the notion. All this time I've worried about dragging myself, with all these intense emotions, to whatever comes after death. How unnecessary!

In this moment during Ruth's funeral I surface out of paralyzing pain toward the living. I've pulled far away from my husband during Ruth's dying time. Suddenly aware of him and his tears for our friend, I lean against my beloved and close my eyes and let the sound of the "Hallelujah Chorus" pour over my being.

I peek through tear-covered eyelashes and see that the diamond in my wedding ring has taken on a glow, a reflection from the rhinestones on my blouse and sunlight. For a few moments I play with the notion that Ruth is sending me one last gift, here at her funeral. I watch with awe as the light from the ring forms a cross that turns a bright shade of red.

"Ruth always loved a little touch of red in every room," Maude had said just last night. The cross formed by light turns green, then blue, and forms two perfect independent hearts.

After the funeral service Maude kisses me goodbye. It is her words of immeasurable pain that draw me back into earth's realities. "Them funeral words were nice," she tells me, "but in the end all we really got was lonely."

God

Forgive me

I
Renounce
&
Reclaim

I
Spit fire
&
Pray

I
Cling
Then
Push away

Today I'm
Lost

Will
I
Ever
Be
Found

Amen.

You know me,
Elizabeth

Chapter Seventeen

Lonely in Heaven

Ruth's family flies back to Tennessee with her body in the airplane. In the days after Ruth's death, my grieving begins to return to anger. Death. I reject that word!

I blame God for taking Ruth's life. Looking straight up to the sky and shaking my fist, I say, "Someone"—meaning God—"made an irresponsible decision." Is there a good and great God, the kind of God that Ruth absolutely believed in? I wonder.

Our lives belong to God. Do I believe that or are they just words? Human words. I want those words to feel true to me.

What if no one's in charge? Could I handle that knowledge and not feel guilty for daring not to believe in God?

The depth of my sadness scares me.

Grief is a natural process. However, the intensity of it can be frightening. Church, where I once found joy, does not seem relevant to me. I don't know if I am repulsed by or envious of people who seem to feel God's presence so clearly.

"It is okay to be angry with God" is not news to me. I have always understood that God would allow for anger. These are human emotions. "God has much to explain, and we can ask him anything we need to know someday," I had been told many years ago.

At Ruth's funeral, when her childhood minister spoke about how people seem to believe there are exact reasons for everything and godly plans for our lives and that "someday God will give us the answers to all these questions that we have," he added, "I suspect that when we die, these earthly questions will not seem necessary. The things that seem important will have no meaning as we know it." Those words are comforting to me. We really do not know anything about life everlasting, do we?

Life is far too fragile. I struggle to believe in Ruth's God, clinging to life and earthly behavior.

Tessie's children are worried. "Do you think that Ms. Ruth might be bored in heaven?" one of them asks. Tessie realizes that her child is afraid that if Ms. Ruth might be bored in heaven, then she might also have time to be lonely in heaven. Heaven to Tessie's children, because she taught them to have such wonderful childlike faith, is so real that they think of heaven as a place where emotions are like those we have here on earth. I think I must have learned to think that way myself.

Paul and Robin think of heaven as a place where they will join Ruth someday. Many of my friends have said to me, "For the first time I am not afraid to die because I know that Ruth is there in heaven. Now I am not afraid to go there."

Maude has a terrible time understanding why God did not heal her beloved child. "I prayed for a miracle and He could have given one. So why didn't he?"

Ruth had told her, "Mama, don't be mad at God. Be mad at cancer."

"Trust and obey, for there's no other way, but to trust and obey . . ." are the words to an old hymn that we learned as children in church so long ago. What if there is no reason to trust?

Trust what—that God will take care of us? My anger and the pain from Ruth's death lock me into an inconsolable mood. Many Sundays I sit in church and in my mind, Ruth's once joyful face now seems to be covered in pain. I focus on the cross hanging on the wall in the sanctuary. Ruth's body is still hanging there, and the vision of those terrible last weeks of Ruth's life will not leave my mind. The dark red blood, the yellow tones of her skin, the deep purple-red bruising. I sit in my favorite pew and remember her smiling face, now stilled, solemn, and lifeless. I imagine her dead body hung on the wooden cross. Here in this church Ruth loved, the image will not leave my mind. I had once found much joy here. My church does not seem relevant to me.

Father

I am dark December
Winter shadows,
Weeping for warmth
Imploring summer's sunlight

Exhausted by questions
Starved for answers
Worn from wear

Lost in empty spaces

Why?

Are
You
Real?

Amen.

Elizabeth

Chapter Eighteen

Closure

Tessie, Sugarbaker, and I sit one morning in a circle on the floor of Ruth's condo with other friends of Ruth's, talking about her a few days after her funeral. We use all the words, the current words about loss and death. Our minister's wife reads the twenty-third Psalm from *The Message,* a contemporary language New Testament.

> Even when the way goes through
> Death Valley,
> I'm not afraid
> when you walk at my side.
> Your trusty shepherd's crook
> makes me feel secure.
> Your beauty and love chase after me
> every day of my life.
> I'm back home in the house of God
> for the rest of my life.

I hope these words are true.

"It is OK to be angry," Tessie says. "Ruth believed in heaven. She is probably trying to tell God a better way to run it. You know she will want Him to organize some Heavenly Sunday school class or some such thing."

We all laugh at Tessie's idea. The cynic in me wonders if God cares about Sunday school classes or any manmade invention of theology. Tessie has a need to believe in this manner.

We take communion that day, using apple juice and cinnamon toast because Sugarbaker and Tessie thought Ruth would like the fact that we borrowed the toast and juice from the children's area of the church. We even bury a little broken-headed Angel under a rose bush near the front door of Ruth's condo. For Tessie and Sugarbaker it is a physical way to say goodbye and it was a remembrance of Ruth. All this is current philosophy for handling death. "Have closure" are the words people use, meaning that everything has a beginning and an ending. Acknowledge your grief and try to move on forward.

It's been months since Ruth was buried. Nothing consoles me. Every time I go to church my eyes are drawn to the brick wall where the large wooden cross hangs. Ruth's still suspended on that church cross, in my mind. When I look at the cross it is as though Ruth is really hanging there, still in her destroyed body, all hollow-eyed, yellowed skin, ruby red-blooded.

Sarah, Ruth's friend who spoke at her funeral months ago, is the visiting speaker at church today. It's all sunshine outside, but my heart still feels gray with grief. I listen as Sarah speaks from the same pulpit from which Ruth often spoke. My eyes are drawn away from the wooden cross to Sarah as she tells a true story about walking outside at dawn one morning and seeing a field covered with bright red poppies. Someone standing next to Sarah in the field clapped his hands. Out of a shimmer of red blossoms, hundreds of yellow butterflies suddenly flew upward. Sarah says she thought, "This is like seeing the face of God."

I turn my eyes back to the cross. The image in my mind of my dead friend's body seems to pull free from the wooden structure. I watch Ruth moving upward and around the room. She is smiling. For the first time in a long while joy overrides the pain of her death. In the way that mystery often works with no real explanation, it just works; grief no longer holds me captive. I, too, am suddenly free.

Then, I think about what Ruth's minister said. His words had so much impact for me at the funeral. "The follies and fallenness of man and mind and earth and body will be reduced to irrelevance."

Whatever happens after death, the same old frightened me, the lost, left-alone child, will not travel that star-covered journey. That part of me will be left behind.

Ruth's lost dreams are not lost at all, only limited by my earthly eyes. Ruth's disappointment, not getting to live out her life, ended at death. Ruth is so far beyond that space where we mortals place our dreams. She does not miss them or long for their completion. Ruth's suffering is over. The intensity of grief can be so frightening that I had forgotten it is a natural process.

I'm different now; I understand there is no reason to fear death. I lean toward my life's pattern, a need to trust in a higher power.

I still wonder at times about all my "what ifs." What if there is no heaven? What if there is no God? It would mean Ruth's life would simply be over, her body turned into dust. Ruth can't be only dust, discarded ash. I don't believe that life, however compelling, is more than what follows life. It wouldn't make sense. A mighty force able to create life will most certainly create *more beyond life*. Death cannot be less than life. There is more.

As a little girl, the moment I first learned to love and be loved there was a natural craving in me to say, "Thank you and amen." Without knowing the words, I trusted the spirit within. It is only the foolish adult in me who has this need to question everything.

I pray and feel soft breezes blowing over glistening red poppies, butterflies flurrying, a colorful dance, all silky red and yellow promises.

I still see myself kneeling, as a small child, counting camellia cuttings growing under jelly jars in damp moss green under an abandoned house. Mother had been rooting the flowers before she got sick. The living, growing plants were my proof beyond memory that my mother lived before she died and left me. I was taught God loves me. I have experienced a lifelong struggle trying to understand an invisible power that allows painful processes to happen and still grants an undeniable mystery of joy in their midst. How could I feel so sad and still be able, at some point, to know gladness?

Ruth's faith was more simplistic than mine. For whatever reason, she was able to love God with passion the same way I find it natural to flush with pleasure at the sight of a flower or have goose bumps come on my arms at the sound of the church choir. Words in hymns don't change anything, but the meanings behind them change everything. Both simplistic faith and complex faith are acceptable extremes of belief. The need to gather evidence of God has taught me but one thing: I know who I am. I was given—He gave me, Elizabeth—a gift for knowing, loving, and creating. How this happened is beyond human knowledge.

Father

My carefully etched map
Leads nowhere.
Your pathways reveal themselves.
Firm stones
Guide the way.
Every loving thing
Clearly points to home.

I love you.

Elizabeth

Part Two

"Reflections"

Prologue

Meditation

What's the price of a pet canary? Some loose change, right? And God cares what happens to it even more than you do. He pays attention to you, down to the last detail—even numbering the hairs on your head! So don't be intimidated by all this bully talk. You're worth more than a million canaries. (from Matthew 10 in *The Message* by Eugene Peterson)

Discussion

His Eye is on the sparrow and He watches over me.

Elizabeth had reason to question God's presence in the world. As a child, did you feel that God watched over your life? What positive and what negative things made your life better or worse based on this idea?

That's the flip side of double-edged knowledge. Maybe Mother didn't know that complete gladness means you can reach just as deeply into the core of life's sadness.

Can a person experience true happiness if she or he knows nothing about sadness? Are things ever as good or as bad as you expect? How would you measure happiness if you had never known sadness?

Does God pick and choose good or bad things to happen to people? Do you believe things happen at random? How do you explain your position?

"Mercy me, Elizabeth. Someday you'll trust your knowledge. God is God. Seeing, feeling, proving—that's Earth-connected stuff."

Are there times when you trust some people's faith more than you trust the faith of others? Why? How did faith play a role in your childhood? Write a short prayer of thanksgiving for one of the people in your life who most helped shape your faith.

Chapter 1

Meditation

Give your entire attention to doing what God is doing right now, and don't get worked up about what may or may not happen tomorrow. God will help you deal with whatever hard things come up when the time comes. (from Matthew 6, *The Message*)

Discussion

"Damn and double damn," she would say, but her innocence belied these words and was part of [Ruth's] charm . . .

Can anyone be all good or all bad? Are people predisposed one way or the other from birth? List five behaviors you define as "good" and five you define as "bad." How are they similar? What makes a behavior good or bad?

Of the people you know, who leans more toward your definition of
"good" and who leans more toward "bad"? How do you respond to
each type of person? Are you able to be aware of both aspects
within someone and still care for her/him?

Which parts of your own personality do you find in conflict with
your idea of the way you want to see yourself?

*[Ruth sings] "There's within my heart a melody. Jesus whispers sweet
and low, fills my every longing, keeps me singing as I go."*

What role does music play in your life? What types of music do you
prefer? What types do you dislike? Why?

Do songs come to mind when you need comfort? If so, what songs?
When did you learn them? If not, what does comfort you?

Chapter 2

Meditation

We are not alone. Earth forms us
past and present, peoples near and far,
*   show us who we are.*
Through a human life God finds us;
dying, living, love is fully known,
and in bread and wine reminds us.
*   We are not our own.*
(from Brian Wren's "We Are Not Our Own" [Carol Stream IL:
Hope Publishing, 1989])

Discussion

Ruth sees past personal veneer, looks into a person's heart, and finds a
spirit's potential.

What importance do you give to a person's formal education and/or
social class in considering her/him a close friend?

Name three friends. If your own circumstances were visibly altered (positively or negatively), would those friends still be there for you? Would you want them as your friends? How would you handle finding out they would not stand by you?

"My Mommy taught me that sin is like soot on snow," Ruth might say. "I crawled under the house the day Mother died," I might answer, "to count the camellias she had been rooting under overturned jelly jars."

Through turbulent childhoods, Ruth and Elizabeth held sustaining beliefs—God is real and accessible. Ruth drew comfort from the things she learned about Christ as a child and trusted Him in spite of the harshness of her life. What did your childhood teach you about God? How did what you were taught about God as a child form the person you became?

It's not unusual to hear Ruth singing to them, "There is no one exactly like you. You can search the whole world over, but there is no one exactly like you."

How do you see yourself? How do others see you? How close are these two images of yourself?

Chapter 3

Meditation

No one so utterly desolate, "…There's a song in every silence, seeking word and melody; there's a dawn in every darkness bringing hope to you and me. From the past will come the future; what it holds, a mystery, unrevealed until its season, something God alone can see…." (from "In the Bulb There Is a Flower," words and music by Natalie Sleeth, copyright 1986)

Then was our mouth filled with laughter, and our tongues with singing. The Lord hath done great things for us, whereof we are glad…. (Psalm 126:2, KJV)

No one is so accursed by fate,
But some heart, though unknown,
Responds to His own.
(Henry Longfellow)

Discussion

[Ruth says] "…I will not be able to bear a child. I wanted to have babies! Even if I live I will never be able to have them. There are so many things left that I want to do. Why, why?"

How many things would you feel you had left undone if you knew your own life were ending? What goals have you set for yourself? What are the reasons you have left any of them undone?

[Ruth says] "Elizabeth, I am going to get French marrow! Call me. The donor lives in Paris. Just think, in this whole wide world, there is someone just for me."

Would you be willing to go through the painful process of being an organ donor for someone you love? Who?

How much difficulty would you have being a donor for a stranger? Why?

Chapter 4

Mediation

My soul counseled me and charged me to seek that which is unseen: and my soul revealed unto me that the thing we grasp is the thing we Desire.... (from *Prose Poems* by Kahlil Gibran)

Discussion

"I must tell Jesus all of my troubles," the voice sings. I look up, and Ruth is walking toward the pulpit...singing.

Ruth's confidence comes from faith. Name someone or something in whom or in which you find that kind of reassurance. Why did you name this person or thing?

Over the weeks I decide to claim the words from Ruth's sermon and place them in the context of my own need.

Words have power. They can harm. They can affirm. What words have brought joy to you? Is there someone who could use a kind word that you have the power to speak?

Chapter 5

Meditation

Friends, when life gets really difficult, don't jump to the conclusion that God isn't on the job. Instead, be glad that you are in the very thick of what Christ experienced. This is a spiritual refining process, with glory just around the corner. (from 1 Peter 4, *The Message*)

Discussion

But I feel unconnected to the laughter and gaiety at the party. It might be Ruth's last birthday.

What if your next birthday were your last? What would you want to be sure to do beforehand? How would you spend it, with whom, and why?

Ruth's love of life demands a chance. The "French Marrow," as we call it, seems to be that opportunity.

Ruth had a choice to live a few years not feeling well or risk a bone marrow transplant and live or die, depending on its success. Which choice might you make if your own life were on the line? Why? What factors in your life would influence your decision?

Chapter 6

Meditation

*What a God we have! And how fortunate we are to have him, this
Father of our Master Jesus! Because Jesus was raised from the dead,
we've been given a brand-new life and have everything to live for,
including a future in heaven—and the future starts now. God is keeping
careful watch over us and the future. The Day is coming when you'll be
all—life healed and whole. (from 1 Peter 1, The Message)*

Discussion

*Her sister has made what they call a bargain with Ruth. Robin said,
"I'll put my life on hold and stay with you and help you every way
possible. You do your part, and together we will get through this transplant."*

For whom would you be willing to put your life "on hold"? Why?
Who would you expect to do as much for you? What if they didn't?

Ruth has developed a fondness for the kind and gentle radiologist, Dr. Keller, who is fascinated that Ruth is an ordained Baptist minister.

Why do some people believe only men are called to be ordained ministers, while others believe women are also called to serve in this manner? What do you believe? How do you respond to people whose beliefs are different from yours regarding gender and ministry?

When I leave to go home, Robin tells me, "Ruth will be all right, I just know it. We'll get our miracle."

Do you believe in miracles? Why?

Chapter 7

Meditation

Everything in the world is about to be wrapped up, so take nothing for granted. Stay wide-awake in prayer. Most of all love each other as if your life depended on it. Love makes up for practically anything . . . . Be generous with the different things God gave you, passing them around so all get in on it: if words, let it be God's words; if help, let it be God's hearty help. That way, God's bright presence will be evident in every-thing through Jesus, and he'll get all the credit as the One mighty in everything—encores to the end of time. Oh yes! (from 1 Peter 4, *The Message*)

Discussion

Sugarbaker gets an inspiration. "Y'all, let's draw huge smiling lips on them before we go inside." Ruth howls when she sees the bright red lipstick lip smiles. "Ruth continues to keep her sense of humor and very pleasant personality," says Paul.

How large a part does humor play in your life? What are some examples where humor made a big difference in your life?

What does humor bring to death and dying?

[Ruth] takes the French marrow in her hands and says, "This is my life, right here. My physical life is in this bag. As I drift off to sleep at some point this night, I am going to imagine that the marrow is a great ocean entering my body, going deeply, deeply into the cave of my bone and that all of it will stay and begin to grow and make new cells to replace all those that were too weak to fight. This is my challenge."

What challenges are the ones you find most difficult? Why?

For the next week, try praying with your hands cupped and held in front of you as you say, "I hold the direction of my life in my hands, Lord. Help me listen for your guidance each day."

Paul comments afterward, "No one talked—we didn't have to. God revealed himself in his servant, Ruth."

In what ways is God revealed in your life?

Can you sense God in silence? If so, how? If not, why?

Are your prayers truly conversations with God or habitual monologues?

Chapter 8

Meditation

Don't ever feel discouraged, for Jesus is your friend;
and if you lack for knowledge he'll not refuse to lend.
There is a balm in Gilead to make the wounded whole.
(from "There Is a Balm in Gilead," African-American Spiritual)

Discussion

"All I really need is a song in my heart, food in my belly, love in my family."

What three things do you really need to be happy and feel your life is complete? Why?

Suddenly my mind is fused with color. All I can see is bright red, strong yellow. I shake my head. No!

What are your physical responses to grief?

Have you given symbolic value to things in times of grief that were not normally important to you (for example, angels, words, colors, etc.)? Are these same things important to you later? Do they give you comfort or painful memories?

"...As we go from here today, may we have the gifts of: the compassion and resourcefulness of the Good Samaritan, the energy of Martha, and the inner peace of Mary. And may we have the wisdom to know when to call upon each of these gifts."

What are your own gifts? How have you offered them to people in need? How can you reinforce the strength of these gifts, which are already part of who you are?

Name one person who has always offered support to you. Take a moment to offer a prayer of thanksgiving for that person in your life. Remember to tell that special person how much she or he means to you.

Chapter 9

Meditation

The word became flesh and blood, and moved into the neighborhood.
(from John 1, *The Message*)

Discussion

Later Sarah tells me, "Ruth is determined to come back to Mississippi. She wants to be with her friends and family now." Then she adds, "I believe she spent today talking to God."

If you knew death was soon, how would you spend your last hours? Who would you want near you? Are there things previously left unsaid that you want to say to people you love?

What prayer would you find yourself saying if you were near death right now? Write it here.

[Elizabeth] This feeling of desertion is something I felt early in my life. Forsaken. Rage at the idea that Ruth is feeling alone fuels flickering flames within my soul.

Are you afraid to deal with death and dying? If so, why?

Is there someone you met in church, work, or socially who is lonely? How could you make a difference in her or his life?

In the eighteen hours before Ruth returns to Mississippi, our church prepares a home for her. We take her furniture out of storage and paint Ruth's new bedroom soft blue, the color she requests. We get a new home ready for her last homecoming in less than a day. Everyone works round-the-clock. It gives each person something to do for Ruth. It's important to surround her with her own belongings, however brief this time.

If you were aware of when your time to die draws near, to what material things would you feel connected and want near you? Why?

Do you cover your grief or helplessness with staying busy? How important is it that you feel useful when you are helpless?

Chapter 10

Meditation

What came into existence was Life,
And the Life was Light to live by.
The Life-Light blazed out of the darkness;
The darkness couldn't put it out.
(from John 1, *The Message*)

Discussion

"I am going to lean hard on you. My family will not be able to bear that I have cancer. You are one of the few people I know who can handle something like this." I remember my promise. "I am strong and I will help you do whatever you must do."

Ruth doesn't hesitate to explain to Elizabeth what needs she can meet. If you were dying, what would be some of your own needs? Could you use the wisdom of Ruth and ask your friends specifically for the kind of support you needed from each of them?

Could you respond to a loved one in whatever way he or she asked? What source of courage would you call on to help you respond appropriately?

What would you be unwilling to do? Would you be able easily to set aside your own self-interest and opinions to meet the other person's needs in the way he or she desires?

Later, after Ruth is settled into her new home, she looks at me and says out of the blue, "You. You are centered." I ask Ruth, "Did you mean self-centered?" "No, I said you are a centered person."

What does it mean to be a centered person? What gifts does being centered bring to a death and dying situation? How centered are you? How do you describe yourself? How do you think others see you?

We surround Ruth with her own earthly belongings she has missed so much in the stark hospital. We show her love in every human manner as we helplessly wait for her death.

Why do Ruth's friends think she needs to be surrounded by her belongings?

Chapter 11

Meditation

This is complex and often misunderstood, but I want you to be informed and knowledgeable . . . . God wants us to use our intelligence, to seek to understand as well as we can . . . . God's various gifts are handed out everywhere; but they all originate in God's Spirit. God's various ministries are carried out everywhere; but they all originate in God's Spirit . . . . Each person is given something to do that shows who God is: Everyone gets in on it, everyone benefits. All kinds of things are handed out by the Spirit, and to all kinds of people! (from 1 Corinthians 12, The Message)

Discussion

[Elizabeth] I mentally divide up this precious time. The first night I call "Show Time," but after that first night I accept we're in "Real Time."

How would you divide and title the segments of your life?

How much of your life is for "show" and how much is spent being true, sincere, and real?

[Elizabeth] But I find myself relishing the miracles that surround Ruth: her passion for life, her utter belief in God.

How would a miracle sound? Taste? Smell? Feel?

What have you experienced that you would define as a miracle in your life? Did it change you? If so, how?

Are there miracles occurring to which you are oblivious because you don't understand how they connect to the present?

Chapter 12

Meditation

All kinds of things are handed out by the Spirit, to all kinds of people!
The variety is wonderful . . . (from 1 Corinthians 12, *The Message*)

But when we have been made perfect and complete, the need for these
inadequate gifts will come to an end, and they will disappear.
(1 Corinthians 13:10, *The Living Bible*, paraphrased)

Some day we are going to see him in his completeness, face to face. Now
all that I know is hazy and blurred, but then I will see everything
clearly, just as clearly as God sees into my heart right now.
(1 Corinthians 13:11 TLB, paraphrased)

There are three things that remain—faith, hope, and love—and the
greatest of these is love. (1 Corinthians 13:13, TLB, paraphrased)

Discussion

The most difficult part of Ruth's dying is that the unfairness of an
early death will leave Ruth with so much living left undone. She
wanted to have children. She had so much to give to the world—so
many spirit-filled gifts to share.

How would you feel if you knew you were dying at the age you are now? How old does a person have to be before you do not consider his or her death an "early death"?

What things have you been able to do with your life that you feel are worthy? List them.

Which of your own gifts would you call spirit-filled? In what ways do you share your abilities, talents, hobbies, and passions with other people?

How can we bear what Ruth must bear? Why would a just God be so unjust?

In the death and dying process of your own loved ones, what losses have been and/or would be the hardest to bear?

What are or have been some of your responses to the feeling that life is unfair? What role does God play in the fairness and unfairness of life?

Can you pray a person well? Can enough folks pray so long and so truly that God will hear them and answer their prayers? Are prayers just empty words, bouncing off walls with no ceilings? Prayer brings the blessing of strength, making it possible to live through whatever you must bear. Prayer can bring peace; it can bring serenity. Can it change or alter the course of death? I don't think so, but sometimes prayers seem to be answered in unexpected moments.

From what resources do you draw strength to move throughout each day?

How much does prayer help you?

Have there been times when you felt that your prayers seemed to be answered in unexpected moments? If so, when? What was your initial response?

How do you handle the answer to your prayers not being the answer you desire?

Chapter 13

Meditation

*My soul counseled me and instructed me to see that the light which I
carry is not my light,*
That my song was not created within me;
For though I travel with the light, I am not the light,
and though I am a lute fastened with strings, I am not the lute-player.
(from *Prose Poems* by Kahlil Gibran)

Discussion

Help in the form of a friend comes to Ruth's front door.

What sources of help have come to you in times of trouble?

Do your prayers change in times of need from the way you pray
when things are going well? Does the frequency of your praying
change?

For one week, say one prayer each day filled only with
thanksgiving.

The trees stagger; their roots burrow deep. They cling like Ruth and me
to earth. I close my eyes and humbly bow my own head. The light is
going out. Darkness is falling.

Elizabeth clings to earthly things. When the chips are down, what
is of real value that you can cling to? What earthly things have
value to you in death and dying?

"Yes," I murmur and whimper inside my head the very words I've most
wanted not to utter. "It is time now. Come, Lord. Take Ruth home."
Hurry, hurry.

At what point of pain and suffering do you think you might choose
to forego additional life-sustaining measures? At what point would
you desire medical treatment to be ended? What influences do your
current age, health, and family situation have on your choices?

Chapter 14

Meditation

Compared to what's coming, living conditions around here seem like a stopover in an unfurnished shack, and we're tired of it! We've been given a glimpse of the real thing, our true home, our resurrection bodies! The Spirit of God whets our appetite by giving us a taste of what's ahead. He puts a little of heaven in our hearts so that we'll never settle for less. (from 2 Corinthians 5, *The Message*)

There I stood gazing at the waves, listening to their singing,
and considering the power that lies behind them—
The power that travels with the storm.
And rages with the volcano, that smiles with smiling flowers and makes
Melody with murmuring brooks . . . .
(from *Revelation* by Kahlil Gibran)

Discussion

[Elizabeth's letter to Ruth] "The phrase 'Life Everlasting' keeps coming into my mind. Life Everlasting, a kind of life that I know nothing about. Do you think that it is possible? Life Everlasting, I mean? I bet you know so much more about that than I do right now."

What does the phrase "life everlasting" mean to you?

[Paul] *"Whoever handles Ruth's body must use absolute tenderness."*

What part of a person do you believe exists beyond death? How would you describe that part of yourself?

[Elizabeth's lament] *"Cure what you've done, Lord. Help us to forgive what you've done . . . Thank you for your girl, Lord."*

Bargaining is considered a common stage of grief. If you begged God to cure someone you love, how would you feel if healing resulted in death instead of life?

Chapter 15

Meditation

Will the Lord cast off forever? And will He be favorable no more?
Is His mercy clean gone forever? Doth His promises fail forever more?
(Psalm 77:7, KJV)

For we know that if our earthly house of this tabernacle were dissolved,
we have a building of God, a house not made with hands, eternal in the
heavens . . .
(2 Corinthians 5:1, KJV)

Discussion

When [Maude] opens the card, many colorful birds jump out and the
message reads, "All the birds in heaven are whistling at you."

Do you feel the presence of loved ones who have died? If so, how
would you describe it? When do you sense them? If not, how do
you interpret the experiences of those who say they do?

Imagine that the inhabitants of heaven watch the living. How would you alter what you do as daily routine if your loved ones could look from heaven and observe you? How would you acknowledge them?

[North Church member to Maude] "The cross is a statement about the nature of God's love. It is the emblem of atonement and the symbol of salvation and redemption through Christianity," says the friend, pointing out the designs on the pall. "The intertwined ovals represent the Trinity—Father, Son, and Holy Spirit. Blue, the color of the sky, symbolizes heaven and heavenly love. It is also the color of truth because blue always appears in the sky after the clouds have disappeared, suggesting the unveiling of truth. These expressions clearly represent all of Ruth's strong beliefs."

These expressions of hope clearly represent Ruth's beliefs. What things in your home are symbolic of the way you live your life? Look around your house and collect five of these symbols. Write a paragraph explaining what each represents in your life.

I walk back into the church sanctuary and sit on my favorite pew. The cross hangs high above the organ on a blank wall. I am horrified to realize that in the past when I looked at this cross I've often felt peace. Now, when I look, shadows fall across the image of the body of Ruth hanging there, a yellow-skinned, blood-covered body of my own disbelief.

Elizabeth's grief is so great that she sees an image of her friend hanging on the church cross. Does faith come easily for you? What role does your faith play during times of intense grief?

Why do some people seem to question everything and others appear to accept everything at face value? Toward which extreme do you lean? Are you more patient with those who lean more one way or the other?

If your own soul were laid bare for the world to see, what would it show about what you believe and why?

Chapter 16

Meditation

They all realized they were in a place of holy mystery, that God was at work among them. They were quietly worshipful—then noisily grateful, calling out among themselves, "God is back, looking to the needs of His people!" (from Luke 7, *The Message*)

There I saw you, night, tragic and beautiful and awesome,
standing between the heaven and the Earth,
with clouds for your garment, girdled with the fog.
(from *Prose Poems* by Kahlil Gibran)

Discussion

"The follies and fallenness of man and mind and earth and body will, in the light of His glory and grace, be reduced to irrelevance." (Dr. Steve Pressley, Ruth's childhood minister)

What part of yourself would you willingly leave behind at death? What part would you most regret putting aside?

How do you honor and keep the memory of the person(s) you love alive and still let go of the darkness of grief?

Chapter 17

Meditation

They were puzzled, wondering what to make of this. Then, out of nowhere it seemed, two men, light cascading over them, stood there. The women were awestruck and bowed down in worship. The men said, "Why are you looking for the Living One in a Cemetery? He is not here, but raised up." (from Luke 24, *The Message*)

In my distress I screamed to the Lord for His help.
And He heard me from heaven; my cry reached His ears.
(Psalm 18:6, TLB, paraphrased)

Discussion

[Elizabeth] Is there a good and great God, the kind of God that Ruth absolutely believed in? I wonder.

How were you taught to express anger? As an adult, how do you allow yourself to be truly angry? Or do you?

Have there been times when you felt angry toward God? Do you allow yourself to rail at God, or do you bury your hurt, anger, and pain as if God is unaware of it? Are you able to release the pain of that anger?

To forgive is to renounce anger or resentment, making a conscious decision not to be punitive. Who does denied and ignored anger punish? How? Write a prayer asking God for help in forgiving.

Ruth had told her, "Mama, don't be mad at God. Be mad at cancer."

What do you believe about why things happen to people? What role do you assign God?

Here in this church Ruth loved, the image will not leave my mind. I had once found much joy here. My church does not seem relevant to me.

Where do you find joy? What things in your life are relevant?

Chapter 18

Meditation

Will the Lord walk off and leave us for good?
Will He never smile again?
Is His love worn threadbare?
Has His salvation promise burned out?
Has God forgotten His Manners?
Has He angrily stalked off and left us?
"Just my luck," I said. "The High God goes out of business
Just the moment I need Him."
(from Psalm 77, *The Message*)

Discussion

Sarah says she thought, "This is like seeing the face of God."

In how many places have you found the face of God?

For the first time in a long while joy overrides the pain of her death. In the way that mystery often works with no real explanation, it just works; grief no longer holds me captive. I, too, am suddenly free.

With what fears do you prefer to live instead of addressing them?
Why?

What if there is no heaven?

Would you live your life in a different manner if you knew there
was no afterlife? Why? If so, how would you live it differently?

*Both simplistic faith and complex faith are acceptable extremes of
belief.*

Do you agree with this statement? Why or why not? List three
simple concepts of faith you were taught as a child. Do you agree
with them now? Why or why not?

How this happened is beyond human knowledge.

How comfortable are you with ambiguity? Is it okay with you to live a lifetime with unanswered questions?

How dependent is your faith on having answered questions?

Prayer Experience
Elizabeth tells God at the end of many of her prayers: *It's me, Elizabeth.* In an honest conversation with God today, how would you identify yourself in limited words?

Write your own prayer. Address God with a name that most expresses what you need today: *Shepherd*, a nurturer and caretaker of humankind; *Lord,* acknowledging God is over all we see and know; *My Heavenly Father*, the One who protects and directs life; or *Spirit*, the breath of life before, now, and beyond death. Include one line in your prayer that asks a question, one line that expresses gratitude, and one line that is not self-oriented.

www.ingramcontent.com/pod-product-compliance
Lightning Source LLC
Chambersburg PA
CBHW062058270326
41931CB00013B/3136